This report contains the collective views of an international group of experts and does not necessarily represent the decisions or the stated policy of the United Nations Environment Programme, the International Labour Organisation, or the World Health Organization.

Environmental Health Criteria 121

ALDICARB

First draft prepared by Dr J. Risher and Dr H. Choudhury, US Environmental Protection Agency, Cincinnati, Ohio, USA

Published under the joint sponsorship of the United Nations Environment Programme, the International Labour Organisation, and the World Health Organization

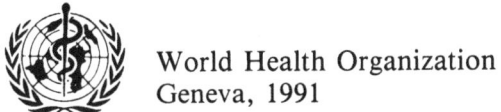

World Health Organization
Geneva, 1991

The **International Programme on Chemical Safety (IPCS)** is a joint venture of the United Nations Environment Programme, the International Labour Organisation, and the World Health Organization. The main objective of the IPCS is to carry out and disseminate evaluations of the effects of chemicals on human health and the quality of the environment. Supporting activities include the development of epidemiological, experimental laboratory, and risk-assessment methods that could produce internationally comparable results, and the development of manpower in the field of toxicology. Other activities carried out by the IPCS include the development of know-how for coping with chemical accidents, coordination of laboratory testing and epidemiological studies, and promotion of research on the mechanisms of the biological action of chemicals.

WHO Library Cataloguing in Publication Data

Aldicarb.

(Environmental health criteria ; 121)

1.Aldicarb - adverse effects   2.Aldicarb - toxicity   3.Environmental exposure   4.Environmental pollutants   I.Series

ISBN 92 4 157121 7   (NLM Classification: WA 240)
ISSN 0250-863X

©World Health Organization 1991

Publications of the World Health Organization enjoy copyright protection in accordance with the provisions of Protocol 2 of the Universal Copyright Convention. For rights of reproduction or translation of WHO publications, in part or *in toto*, application should be made to the Office of Publications, World Health Organization, Geneva, Switzerland. The World Health Organization welcomes such applications.

The designations employed and the presentation of the material in this publication do not imply the expression of any opinion whatsoever on the part of the Secretariat of the World Health Organization concerning the legal status of any country, territory, city, or area or of its authorities, or concerning the delimitation of its frontiers or boundaries.

The mention of specific companies or of certain manufacturers' products does not imply that they are endorsed or recommended by the World Health Organization in preference to others of a similar nature that are not mentioned. Errors and omissions excepted, the names of proprietary products are distinguished by initial capital letters.

PRINTED IN FINLAND
Vammalan Kirjapaino Oy
91/8809 — VAMMALA — 5200

CONTENTS

ENVIRONMENTAL HEALTH CRITERIA FOR ALDICARB

1. SUMMARY 11
   1.1 Identity, properties, and analytical methods 11
   1.2 Uses, sources, and levels of exposure 11
   1.3 Kinetics and metabolism 12
   1.4 Studies on experimental animals 13
   1.5 Effects on humans 13

2. IDENTITY, PHYSICAL AND CHEMICAL PROPERTIES, AND ANALYTICAL METHODS 14
   2.1 Identity 14
   2.2 Physical and chemical properties 14
   2.3 Conversion factors 15
   2.4 Analytical methods 15

3. SOURCES OF HUMAN AND ENVIRONMENTAL EXPOSURE 20
   3.1 Natural occurrence 20
   3.2 Anthropogenic sources 20
       3.2.1 Production levels, processes, and uses 20
             3.2.1.1 World production figures 21
             3.2.1.2 Manufacturing processes 21

4. ENVIRONMENTAL TRANSPORT, DISTRIBUTION, AND TRANSFORMATION 22
   4.1 Transport and distribution between media 22
       4.1.1 Air 22
       4.1.2 Water and soil 23
       4.1.3 Vegetation and wildlife 35
   4.2 Biotransformation 36
   4.3 Interaction with other physical, chemical or biological factors 38
       4.3.1 Soil microorganisms 38

5. ENVIRONMENTAL LEVELS AND HUMAN EXPOSURE 39
   5.1 Environmental levels 39
       5.1.1 Air 39
       5.1.2 Water 39

	5.1.3 Food and feed	41
5.2	General population exposure	43
5.3	Occupational exposure during manufacture, formulation or use	44

6. KINETICS AND METABOLISM ... 45

   6.1 Absorption ... 45
   6.2 Distribution ... 46
   6.3 Metabolic transformation ... 47
   6.4 Elimination and excretion in expired air, faeces, and urine ... 48

7. EFFECTS ON LABORATORY MAMMALS AND *IN VITRO* TEST SYSTEMS ... 52

   7.1 Single exposure ... 52
   7.2 Short-term exposure ... 54
   7.3 Skin and eye irritation; sensitization ... 57
   7.4 Long-term exposure ... 58
   7.5 Reproduction, embryotoxicity, and teratogenicity ... 58
   7.6 Mutagenicity and related end-points ... 61
   7.7 Carcinogenicity ... 63
   7.8 Other special studies ... 65
   7.9 Factors modifying toxicity; toxicity of metabolites ... 67
   7.10 Mechanisms of toxicity - mode of action ... 67

8. EFFECTS ON HUMANS ... 69

   8.1 General population exposure ... 69
      8.1.1 Acute toxicity; poisoning incidents ... 69
      8.1.2 Human studies ... 71
      8.1.3 Epidemiological studies ... 72
   8.2 Occupational exposure ... 73
      8.2.1 Acute toxicity; poisoning incidents ... 73
      8.2.2 Effects of short- and long-term exposure; epidemiological studies ... 74

9. EFFECTS ON OTHER ORGANISMS IN THE LABORATORY AND FIELD ... 75

   9.1 Microorganisms ... 75
   9.2 Aquatic organisms ... 75
   9.3 Terrestrial organisms ... 78
   9.4 Population and ecosystem effects ... 82

10. EVALUATION OF HUMAN HEALTH RISKS AND EFFECTS ON THE ENVIRONMENT	84
10.1 Evaluation of human health risks	84
10.1.1 Exposure levels	84
10.1.1.1 General population	84
10.1.1.2 Occupational exposure	85
10.1.2 Toxic effects	85
10.1.3 Risk evaluation	86
10.2 Evaluation of effects on the environment	87
11. CONCLUSIONS AND RECOMMENDATIONS	88
11.1 Conclusions	88
11.1.1 General population	88
11.1.2 Occupational exposure	88
11.1.3 Environmental effects	88
11.2 Recommendations	89
12. FURTHER RESEARCH	90
13. PREVIOUS EVALUATIONS BY INTERNATIONAL BODIES	91
REFERENCES	92
RESUME	109
EVALUATION DES RISQUES POUR LA SANTE HUMAINE ET DES EFFETS SUR L'ENVIRONNEMENT	112
CONCLUSIONS ET RECOMMENDATIONS	117
RECHERCHES A EFFECTUER	119
RESUMEN	120
EVALUACION DE LOS RIESGOS PARA LA SALUD HUMANA Y DE LOS EFFECTOS EN EL MEDIO AMBIENTE	123
CONCLUSIONES Y RECOMENDACIONES	128
OTRAS INVESTIGACIONES	130

WHO TASK GROUP ON ENVIRONMENTAL HEALTH CRITERIA FOR ALDICARB

Members

Dr I. Boyer, The Mitre Corporation, McLean, Virginia, USA

Dr G. Burin, Health Effects Division, Office of Pesticide Programs, US Environmental Protection Agency, Washington, DC, USA *(Joint Rapporteur)*

Dr S. Dobson, Institute of Terrestrial Ecology, Monks Wood Experimental Station, Abbots Ripton, Huntingdon, United Kingdom *(Vice Chairman)*

Professor W. J. Hayes, Jr., School of Medicine, Vanderbilt University, Nashville, Tennessee, USA *(Chairman)*

Professor F. Kaloyanova, Institute of Hygiene and Occupational Health, Medical Academy, Sofia, Bulgaria

Dr S. K. Kashyap, National Institute of Occupational Health, Indian Council of Medical Research, Meghani Nagar, Ahmedabad, India

Dr H. P. Misra, University Center for Toxicology, Virginia Polytechnic Institute and State University, Blacksburg, Virginia, USA

Mr D. Renshaw, Department of Health, Hannibal House, London, United Kingdom

Dr J. Withey, Environmental & Occupational Toxicology Division, Environmental Health Center, Tunney's Pasture, Ottawa, Ontario, Canada

Dr Shou-zheng Xue, School of Public Health, Shanghai Medical University, Shanghai, China

Representatives of other organizations

Dr L. Hodges, International Group of National Associations of Manufacturers of Agrochemical Products (GIFAP), Brussels, Belgium

Dr J. M. Charles, International Group of National Associations of Manufacturers of Agrochemical Products (GIFAP), Brussels, Belgium

Secretariat

Dr B. H. Chen, International Programme on Chemical Safety, World Health Organization, Geneva, Switzerland *(Secretary)*

Dr H. Choudhury, Environmental Criteria and Assessment Office, US Environmental Protection Agency, Cincinnati, Ohio, USA *(Joint Rapporteur)*

Dr P. G. Jenkins, International Programme on Chemical Safety, World Health Organization, Geneva, Switzerland

NOTE TO READERS OF THE CRITERIA MONOGRAPHS

Every effort has been made to present information in the criteria documents as accurately as possible without unduly delaying their publication. In the interest of all users of the environmental health criteria monographs, readers are kindly requested to communicate any errors that may have occurred to the Manager of the International Programme on Chemical Safety, World Health Organization, Geneva, Switzerland, in order that they may be included in corrigenda, which will appear in subsequent volumes.

* * *

A detailed data profile and a legal file can be obtained from the International Register of Potentially Toxic Chemicals, Palais des Nations, 1211 Geneva 10, Switzerland (Telephone No. 7988400 or 7985850).

ENVIRONMENTAL HEALTH CRITERIA FOR ALDICARB

A WHO Task Group on Environmental Health Criteria for Aldicarb met in Cincinnati, USA, from 6 to 10 August 1990. Dr C. DeRosa opened the meeting on behalf of the US Environmental Protection Agency. Dr B.H. Chen of the International Programme on Chemical Safety (IPCS) welcomed the participants on behalf of the Manager, IPCS, and the three IPCS cooperating organizations (UNEP/ILO/WHO). The Task Group reviewed and revised the draft criteria monograph and made an evaluation of the risks for human health and the environment from exposure to aldicarb.

The first draft of this monograph was prepared by Dr J. Risher and Dr H. Choudhury of the US Environmental Protection Agency. The second draft was prepared by Dr H. Choudhury incorporating comments received following the circulation of the first draft to the IPCS Contact Points for Environmental Health Criteria documents. During the Task Group meeting all the participants contributed to review the large amount of information submitted by Rhône-Poulenc, and undertook a substantial revision of the second draft. Dr B.H. Chen and Dr P.G. Jenkins, both members of the IPCS Central Unit, were responsible for the overall scientific content and technical editing, respectively.

The efforts of all who helped in the preparation and finalization of the document are gratefully acknowledged. The Secretariat wishes to thank Dr S. Dobson and Dr G. Burin for the significant contributions and revisions of the draft document during the meeting.

Financial support for the meeting was provided by the US Environmental Protection Agency, Cincinnati, USA.

ABBREVIATIONS

ADI	acceptable daily intake
ai	active ingredient
CHO	Chinese hamster ovary
FAD	flavin adenine dinucleotide
FPD	flame photometric detector
GC	gas chromatography
GPC	gel permeation chromatography
HPLC	high-performance liquid chromatography
LC	liquid chromatography
MATC	maximum acceptable toxic concentration
MS	mass spectroscopy
NADPH	reduced nicotinamide adenine dinucleotide phosphate
NOEL	no-observed-effect level
TLC	thin-layer chromatography
UV	ultraviolet

1. SUMMARY

1.1 Identity, properties, and analytical methods

Aldicarb is a carbamate ester. It is a white crystalline solid, moderately soluble in water, and susceptible to oxidation and hydrolytic reactions.

Several different analytical methods, including thin-layer chromatography, gas chromatography (electron capture, flame ionization, etc.), and liquid chromatography, are available. The currently preferred method for analysing aldicarb and its major decomposition products is high-performance liquid chromatography with post-column derivatization and fluorescence detectors.

1.2 Uses, sources, and levels of exposure

Aldicarb is a systemic pesticide that is applied to the soil to control certain insects, mites, and nematodes. The soil application includes a wide range of crops, such as bananas, cotton, coffee, maize, onions, citrus fruits, beans (dried), pecans, potatoes, peanuts, soybeans, sugar beets, sugar cane, sweet potatoes, sorghum, tobacco, as well as ornamental plants and tree nurseries. Exposure of the general population to aldicarb and its toxic metabolites (the sulfoxide and sulfone) occurs mainly through food. The ingestion of contaminated food has led to poisoning incidents from aldicarb and its toxic metabolites (the sulfoxide and sulfone).

Due to the high acute toxicity of aldicarb, both inhalation and skin contact under occupational exposure conditions may be dangerous for workers if preventive measures are inadequate. There have been a few incidents of accidental exposure of workers due to improper use or lack of protective measures.

Aldicarb is oxidized fairly rapidly to the sulfoxide, 48% conversion of parent compound to sulfoxide occurring within 7 days after application to certain types of soils. It is oxidized much more slowly to the sulfone. Hydrolysis of the carbamate ester group, which inactivates the pesticide, is ph dependent, half-lives in distilled water

Summary

varying from a few minutes at a pH of > 12 to 560 days at a pH of 6.0. Half-lives in surface soils are approximately 0.5 to 3 months and in the saturated zone from 0.4 to 36 months Aldicarb hydrolyses somewhat more slowly than either the sulfoxide or the sulfone. Laboratory measurement of the biotic and abiotic breakdown of aldicarb have yielded very variable results and have led to extrapolations radically different from field observation. Field data on the breakdown products of aldicarb furnish more reliable estimates of its fate.

Sandy soils with low organic matter content allow the greatest leaching, particularly where the water table is high. Drainage aquifers and local shallow wells have been contaminated with aldicarb sulfoxide and sulfone; levels have generally ranged between 1 and 50 μg/litre, although an occasional level of approximately 500 μg/litre has been recorded.

As aldicarb is systemic in plants, residues may occur in foods. Residue levels greater than 1 mg/kg have been reported in raw potatoes. In the USA, where the tolerance limit for potatoes is 1 mg/kg, residue levels of up to 0.82 mg/kg have been reported from controlled field trials using application rates recommended by the manufacturer. An upper 95th percentile level of 0.43 mg/kg has been estimated from field trial data, and upper 95th percentile levels of up to 0.0677 mg/kg in raw potatoes have been determined from a market-basket survey.

1.3 Kinetics and metabolism

Aldicarb is efficiently absorbed from the gastrointestinal tract and, to a lesser extent, through the skin. It could be readily absorbed by the respiratory tract if dust were present. It distributes to all tissues, including those of the developing rat fetus. It is metabolically transformed to the sulfoxide and the sulfone (both of which are toxic), and is detoxified by hydrolysis to oximes and nitriles. The excretion of aldicarb and its metabolites is rapid and primarily via the urine. A minor part is also subject to biliary elimination and, consequently, to enterohepatic recycling. Aldicarb does not accumulate in the body as a result of long-term exposure. The inhibition of cholinesterase activity *in vitro* by aldicarb is spontaneously reversible, the half-life being 30-40 min.

1.4 Studies on experimental animals

Aldicarb is a potent inhibitor of cholinesterases and has a high acute toxicity. Recovery from its cholinergic effects is spontaneous and complete within 6 h, unless death intervenes. There is no substantial evidence to indicate that aldicarb is teratogenic, mutagenic, carcinogenic, or immunotoxic.

Birds and small mammals have been killed as a result of ingesting aldicarb granules not fully incorporated into the soil as recommended. In laboratory tests, aldicarb is acutely toxic to aquatic organisms. There is no indication, however, that effects would occur in the field.

1.5 Effects on humans

The inhibition of acetylcholinesterase at the nervous synapse and myoneural junction is the only recognized effect of aldicarb in humans and is similar to the action of organophosphates. The carbamyolated enzyme is unstable, and spontaneous reactivation is relatively rapid compared with that of a phosphorylated enzyme. Non-fatal poisoning in man is rapidly reversible. Recovery is aided by the administration of atropine.

2. IDENTITY, PHYSICAL AND CHEMICAL PROPERTIES, AND ANALYTICAL METHODS

2.1 Identity

Common name: Aldicarb

Chemical structure:

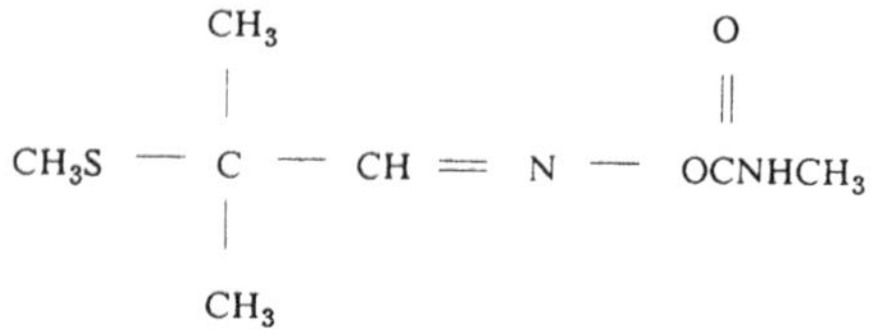

$$CH_3S - \underset{\underset{CH_3}{|}}{\overset{\overset{CH_3}{|}}{C}} - CH = N - O\overset{\overset{O}{\|}}{C}NHCH_3$$

Molecular formula: $C_7H_{14}N_2O_2S$

Synonyms and common trade names: Aldicarb (English); Aldicarbe (French); Carbanolate; ENT 27 093; 2-methyl-2-(methylthio)propanal O-[(methylamino)-carbonyl]oxime (C.A.); 2-methyl-2-(methylthio)propionaldehyde O-methyl-carbamoyloxime (IUPAC); NCI-CO8640; OMS-771; Propanal, 2-methyl-2-(methylthio)-, O-((methylamino)carbonyl)oxime; Temic; Temik; Temik G; Temik M; Temik LD; Sentry; Temik 5G; Temik 10G; Temik 15G; Temik 150G; Union Carbide UC 21 149.

CAS registry number: 116-06-3

RTECS no.: UE2275000.

2.2 Physical and chemical properties

Some physical and chemical properties of aldicarb are given in Table 1.

Aldicarb, for which the IUPAC name is 2-methyl-2-(methylthio)propionaldehyde O-methylcarbamoyloxime, is an oxime carbamate insecticide that was introduced in 1965 by the Union Carbide Corporation under the code number UC 21 149 and the trade name Temik (Worthing & Walker, 1987).

Takusagawa & Jacobson (1977) reported that the molecular structure of the aldicarb crystal, as determined by single-crystal X-ray diffraction techniques, consists of an orthorhombic unit cell with eight molecules per cell. The C-O single bond length in the carbamate group was reported to be significantly greater than in carboxylic acid esters. This supports the theory that interaction with acetylcholinesterase involves disruption of this bond.

Aldicarb has two geometrical isomers as shown below:

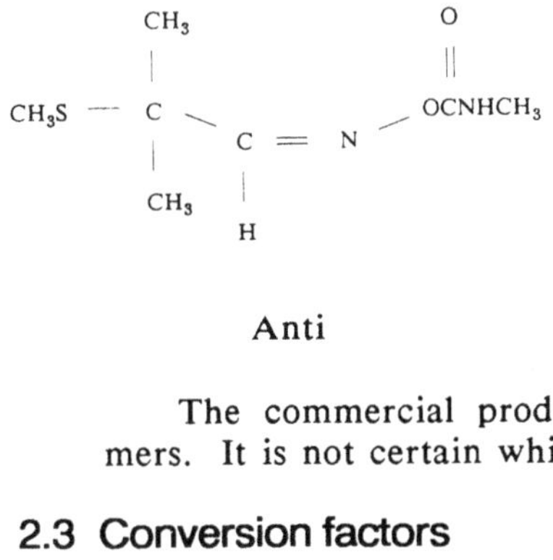

```
      CH₃          O                   CH₃
       |           ||                    |                    O
CH₃S — C           OCNHCH₃      CH₃S — C                      ||
       |  C = N                         |  C = N              OCNHCH₃
      CH₃ |                            CH₃ |
           H                                H

          Anti                              Syn
```

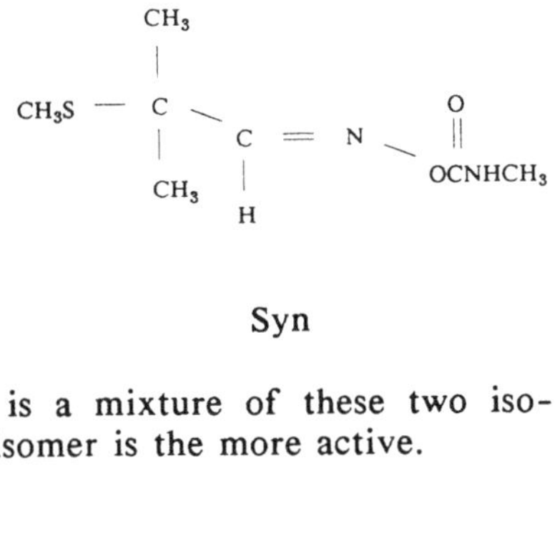

The commercial product is a mixture of these two isomers. It is not certain which isomer is the more active.

2.3 Conversion factors

In air at 25 °C and 101.3 kPa (760 mmHg):

1 ppm (v/v) = 7.78 mg/m^3
1 mg/m^3 = 0.129 ppm (v/v).

2.4 Analytical methods

The methods for analysing aldicarb include thin-layer chromatography (Knaak et al., 1966a,b; Metcalf et al., 1966), liquid chromatography (LC) (Wright et al., 1982), ultraviolet detection (Sparacino et al., 1973), post-column derivatization and fluorometric detection (Moye et al., 1977; Krause, 1979), and gas chromatography (GC) with

Identity, Physical and Chemical Properties, and Analytical Methods

Table 1. Some physical and chemical properties of aldicarb[a]

Relative molecular mass:	190.3
Form:	colourless crystals (odourless or slight sulfurous smell)
Melting point:	100 °C
Boiling point:	unknown; decomposes above 100 °C
Vapour pressure (25 °C):	13 mPa (1 × 10^{-4} mmHg)
Relative density (25 °C):	1.195
Solubility (20 °C):	6 g/litre of water; 40% in acetone; 35% in chloroform; 10% in toluene
Properties:	heat sensitive, relatively unstable chemical; stable in acidic media but decomposes rapidly in alkaline media; non-corrosive to metal; non-flammable; oxidizing agents rapidly convert it to the sulfoxide and slowly to the sulfone
Impurities	dimethylamine; 2-methyl-2-(methylthio) propionitrile; 2-methyl-2-(2-methylthiopropylenaminoxy) propinaldehyde O-(methylcarbamoyl) oxime; 2-methyl-2-(methylthio) propionaldehyde oxime
Log octanol/water partition coefficient	1.359

[a] From: Kuhr & Dorough (1976), Worthing & Walker (1987), and FAO/WHO (1980).

various detectors. These include the Hall detector (Galoux et al., 1979), mass spectrometry (Muszkat & Aharonson, 1983), flame ionization detection (Knaak et al., 1966a,b), and esterification and electron capture detection (Moye, 1975). A multiple residue method exists for detecting N-methylcarbamate insecticide in grapes and potatoes. It involves separation by reverse phase liquid chromatography and detection by a post-column fluorometric technique (AOAC, 1990).

Because of aldicarb's thermal lability, it degrades rapidly in the injection port or on the column during GC analysis. Thus, short columns have been used to facilitate more rapid analyses and prevent thermal degradation (Riva & Carisano, 1969). A major drawback to using GC methods is that aldicarb degrades to aldicarb nitrile during GC; this degradation may also occur in the environment (US EPA, 1984). During GC analysis by conventional-length columns, aldicarb nitrile interferes with aldicarb analysis, thus necessitating a time-consuming clean-up procedure. Furthermore, aldicarb nitrile cannot be detected by LC with UV detection since absorption does not occur in the UV range (US EPA, 1984). The post-column fluorometric technique used in LC requires hydrolysis of the analyte, with the formation of methylamine, which reacts with o-phthalaldehyde to form a fluorophore. Since aldicarb nitrile does not hydrolyse to form methylamine, it cannot be detected (Krause, 1985a).

US EPA (1984) reported that high-performance liquid chromatography (HPLC) can be used to determine N-methylcarbamoyloximes and N-methylcarbamates in drinking-water. With this method, the water sample is filtered and a 400-μl aliquot is injected into a reverse-phase HPLC column. Compounds are separated by using gradient elution chromatography. After elution from the column, the compounds are hydrolysed with sodium hydroxide. The methylamine formed during hydrolysis reacts with o-phthalaldehyde (OPA) to form a fluorescent derivative, which is detected with a fluorescence detector. The estimated detection limit for this method is 1.3 μg aldicarb/litre.

Reding (1987) suggested that samples be kept chilled, acidified with hydrochloric acid to pH 3, and dechlorinated with sodium thiosulfate. Other procedures used were the same as those described in the previous paragraph.

In a collaborative study, Krause (1985a,b) reported an LC multi-residue method for determining the residues of N-methylcarbamate insecticides in crops. The average recovery for 11 carbamates (which included aldicarb and aldicarb sulfone) from 14 crops was 99%, with a coefficient of variation of 8% (fortification levels of 0.03-1.8 mg/kg), and for aldicarb sulfoxide, a very polar metabolite, was 55% and 57% at levels of 0.95 and 1.0 mg/kg, respectively. Methanol and a mechanical ultrasonic homogenizer were used to extract the carbamates. Water-soluble plant co-extractives and non-polar plant lipid materials were removed from the carbamate residues by liquid-liquid partitioning. Additional crop co-extractives (carotenes, chlorophylls) were removed with a Nuchar S-N-silanized Celite column. The carbamate residues were then separated on a reverse-phase LC column, using acetonitrile-water gradient mobile phase. Eluted residues were detected by an in-line post-column fluorometric detection technique. Six laboratories participated in this collaborative study. Each laboratory determined all the carbamates at two levels (0.05 and 0.5 mg/kg) in blind duplicate samples of grapes and potatoes. Repeatability coefficients of variation and reproducibility coefficients of variation for all carbamates in the two crops averaged 4.7 and 8.7%, respectively. The estimated limit of quantification was 0.01 mg/kg.

Ting & Kho (1986) discussed a rapid analytical method using HPLC. They modified their previous method (Ting et al., 1984) by using a 25-cm CH-Cyclohexyl column instead of the 15-cm C-18 column. This modification resulted in the separation of the interference peak found in watermelon co-extractives. The separation of the interference peak and the aldicarb sulfoxide peak was made possible by the additional 10 cm in the length of the column and the higher polarity of the CH-Cyclohexyl. Acetonitrile and methanol were used in the extraction and derivatization procedure before the HPLC determination. Water melons fortified with aldicarb sulfoxide at 0.1, 0.2, and 0.4 mg/kg showed a mean recovery of 74-76%.

Chaput (1988) described a simplified method for determining seven N-methylcarbamates (aldicarb, carbaryl, carbofuran, methiocarb, methomyl, oxamyl, and propoxur) and three related metabolites (aldicarb sulfoxide, aldicarb sulfone, and 3-hydroxy-carbofuran) in fruits and vegetables. Residues are extracted from crops with methanol, and co-extractives are then separated by gel permeation chromatography (GPC) or GPC with on-line Nuchar-Celite clean-up for crops with high chlorophyll and/or carotene content (e.g., cabbage and broccoli). Carbamates are separated on a reverse-phase liquid chromatography column, using a methanol-water gradient mobile phase. Separation is followed by post-column hydrolysis to yield methylamine and by the formation of a flurophore with o-phthalaldehyde and 2-mercaptoethanol prior to fluorescence detection. Recovery data were obtained by fortifying five different crops (apples, broccoli, cabbages, cauliflower, and potatoes) at 0.05 and 0.5 mg/kg. Recoveries averaged 93% at both fortification levels, except in the case of the very polar aldicarb sulfoxide for which recoveries averaged around 52% at both levels. The coefficient of variation of the method at both levels was < 5% and the limit of detection, defined as five times the baseline noise, varied between 5 and 10 µg/kg, depending on the compound.

The International Register of Potentially Toxic Chemicals (IRPTC, 1989) reported a GLC-FPD method for aldicarb analysis in foodstuffs. The limit of quantification was 0.01-0.03 mg/kg with a recovery rate of 76-125%. In this method, the acetone/dichloromethane-extracted sample is evaporated to dryness and the residue is dissolved in a buffered solution of potassium permanganate in water in order to oxidize the thioether pesticide and its sulfoxide metabolite to the corresponding sulfone. Aldicarb sulfone is then extracted with dichloromethane and the extract is evaporated to dryness. The residue is dissolved in acetone and the solution is analysed by GC-FPD using a pyrex column filled with 5% ov-225 on chromosorb W-HP, 150-180 U (the column temperature is 175 °C and the carrier gas is nitrogen with a flow rate of 60 ml/min).

3. SOURCES OF HUMAN AND ENVIRONMENTAL EXPOSURE

3.1 Natural occurrence

Aldicarb is a synthetic insecticide; there are no natural sources of this ester.

3.2 Anthropogenic sources

3.2.1 Production levels, processes, and uses

Aldicarb is a systemic pesticide used to control certain insects, mites, and nematodes. It is applied below the soil surface (either placed directly into the seed furrow or banded in the row) to be absorbed by the plant roots. Owing to the potential for dermal absorption of carbamate insec-ticides (Maibach et al., 1971), aldicarb is produced only in a granular form. The commercial formulation, Temik, is available as Temik 5G, Temik 10G, and Temik 15G, which contain 50, 100, and 150 g aldicarb/kg dry weight, respectively. The metabolite aldicarb sulfone is also used as a pesticide under the common name aldoxycarb. Aldicarb is usually applied to the soil in the form of Temik 5G, 10G, or 15G granules at rates of 0.56-5.6 kg ai/ha. Soil moisture is essential for its release from the granules, and uptake by plants is rapid. Plant protec-tion can last up to 12 weeks (Worthing & Walker, 1987), but actual insecticidal activity may vary from 2 to 15 weeks, depending on the organism involved and on the application method (Hopkins & Taft, 1965; Cowan et al., 1966; Davis et al., 1966; Ridgway et al., 1966). The effective life of this insecticide will vary, depending on the type of soil, the soil moisture, the soil temperature, the rainfall and irrigation conditions, and the presence of soil micro-organisms.

Aldicarb is approved for use on a variety of crops, which include bananas, cotton plants, citrus fruits, coffee, maize, onions, sugar beet, sugar cane, potatoes, sweet potatoes, peanuts, pecans, beans (dried), soybeans, and ornamental plants (FAO/WHO 1980; Berg, 1981). Its use in the home and garden has been proscribed by the manufacturer.

Since aldicarb is used in a granular form, this reduces the handling hazards, as water is necessary for the active ingredient to be released. Respirators and protective clothing should, however, be used in certain field application settings (Lee & Ransdell, 1984).

3.2.1.1 World production figures

In the USA, a total of 725 tonnes was sold domestically for commercial use in 1974 (SRI, 1984).

The US EPA (1985) estimated that aldicarb production from 1979 to 1981 ranged from 1360 to 2130 tonnes/year. In 1988, the US EPA estimated that between 2359 and 2586 tonnes of aldicarb were applied annually in the USA (US EPA, 1988a). More recent world production figures are not available.

3.2.1.2 Manufacturing processes

Aldicarb is produced in solution by the reaction of methyl isocyanate with 2-methyl-2-(methylthio)propanal-doxime (Payne et al., 1966). During normal production, loss to the environment is not significant.

4. ENVIRONMENTAL TRANSPORT, DISTRIBUTION, AND TRANSFORMATION

4.1 Transport and distribution between media

The fate and transport of aldicarb and its decomposition products in various types of soil have been studied extensively under laboratory and field conditions. Owing to the physical properties of aldicarb such as its low vapour pressure, its commercial granular form, and its application beneath the surface of the soil, the vapour hazard of aldicarb is low. Thus the fate of aldicarb in the atmosphere has not received much attention. Similarly, its fate in surface water has not been extensively studied. However, the rates and mechanisms of the hydrolysis of aldicarb have been studied in the laboratory in some detail.

4.1.1 Air

No studies on the stability or migration of aldicarb in the air over or near treated fields have been reported. Laboratory migration studies with radiolabelled aldicarb in various soil types showed a loss of the applied substrate. This loss could not be explained unless aldicarb or its decomposition products had been transferred to the vapour phase (Coppedge et al., 1977). When 34 mg of ^{14}C-aldicarb granules was applied 38 mm below the surface of a column of soil contained in a 63 x 128 mm polypropylene tube, about 43% of the radiolabel was collected in the atmosphere above the column. Additional experiments showed that the transfer of radioactivity to the surrounding atmosphere was inversely proportional to the depth of application in the soil. When ^{14}C- and ^{35}S-labelled aldicarb were used separately in similar experiments, only the experiments in which the ^{14}C-labelled compound was used led to a transfer of radioactivity to the surrounding atmosphere, thus showing that the volatile compound was a carbon-containing breakdown product rather than aldicarb *per se*.

In a subsequent study with aldicarb using ^{14}C at the *S*-methyl, *N*-methyl, and tertiary carbon, Richey et al. (1977) reported that 83% of the radiolabel was recovered as carbon dioxide from a column of soil. The rate of degradation depended on the characteristics of the soil, e.g., pH and humidity.

Supak et al. (1977) reported that when aldicarb (1 mg/g) was applied to clay soil and placed in a volatilizer, its volatilization was very limited. The authors stated that the possibility of aldicarb causing an air contamination hazard when it is applied in the field is negligible since it is applied at a rate of only 1.1-3.4 kg/ha and is inserted to 5-10 cm below the soil surface.

4.1.2 Water and soil

There have been numerous studies on aldicarb, under field and laboratory conditions, to investigate its movement through soil and water, persistence, and degradation. While earlier studies suggested that aldicarb degraded readily in soil and did not leach, later identification of residues in wells indicated that persistence could be longer than predicted and that mobility was greater. Laboratory studies have given variable results and the only totally reliable data are from full-scale field studies.

In one of the few studies conducted with natural water (Quraishi, 1972), rain overflow and seepage water were collected from ditches near untreated fields, filtered, and then treated with aldicarb at a concentration of 100 mg/litre. Solutions were stored in ambient lighting at temperatures ranging from 16 to 20 °C. It took 46 weeks for the aldicarb concentration to decrease to 0.37 mg/litre.

Following an extensive study under laboratory-controlled conditions, Given & Dierberg (1985) reported that the hydrolysis of aldicarb was dependent on pH. They found that the apparent first-order hydrolysis rate over the pH range 6-8 and at 20 °C was relatively slow (Table 2). Above pH 8 the increase in the hydrolysis rate showed a first-order dependence on hydroxide ion concentration. The authors stated that these studies probably represented a "worst-case" situation with respect to the persistence of aldicarb in water, since other means of aldicarb removal or decomposition (e.g., volatilization, adsorption,

Table 2. Apparent first-order rate constant (k), half-life ($t_{1/2}$), and coefficient of variation of the regression line (r^2) for aldicarb hydrolysis at 20 °C in pH-buffered distilled water[a]

pH	Period (days)	k (day^{-1})[b]	$t_{1/2}$[b] (days)	r^2
3.95	89	5.3×10^{-3}	131	0.86
6.02	89	1.2×10^{-3}	559	0.90
7.96	89	2.1×10^{-3}	324	0.62
8.85	89	1.3×10^{-3}	55	0.98
9.85	15	1.2×10^{-1}	6	1.00

[a] Adapted from Given & Dierberg (1985).
[b] Rates and resulting half-life values for pH 6-8 represent only estimates since the slopes of the log percentage remaining versus time regression lines were probably not significantly different from zero.

leaching, and plant and microbial uptake) had been prevented.

Hansen & Spiegel (1983) showed that aldicarb hydrolyses at much slower rates than aldicarb sulfoxide and aldicarb sulfone. Since aldicarb oxidizes fairly rapidly to the sulfoxide and at a slower rate to the sulfone, and subsequent hydrolysis of the oxidation products usually occurs, aldicarb does not persist in the aerobic environment.

In his review, de Haan (1988) discussed leaching of aldicarb to surface water in the Netherlands. Some of the factors favourable to leaching are weak soil binding, high rainfall, irrigation practices, and low transformation rates of the oxidation products of aldicarb.

Aharonson et al. (1987) reported that hydrolysis of aldicarb is one of the abiotic chemical reactions that is linked to the detection of the pesticide in the ground water. The hydrolysis half-life at pH 7 and 15 °C has been estimated by these authors to be as long as 50-500 weeks.

The products of aldicarb hydrolysis at 15 °C under alkaline conditions (pH 12.9 and 13.4) are aldicarb oxime, methylamine, and carbonate (Lemley & Zhong, 1983). The half-lives of hydrolysis at these two pHs are 4.0 and 1.3

min, respectively. Other hydrolysis data, determined at pH 8.5 and 8.2, yielded rates with half-lives of 43 and 69 days, respectively (Hansen & Spiegel, 1983; Krause, 1985a). Lemley et al. (1988) reported that at pH values of 5-8 the sorption of aldicarb, aldicarb sulfoxide, and aldicarb sulfone decreases as the temperature increases from 15 to 35 °C.

Andrawes et al. (1967) applied the pesticide at the recommended rate of 3.4 kg/ha to potato fields and found that < 0.5% of the original dose remained at the end of a 90-day period. In fallow soil, decomposition of aldicarb to its sulfoxide and sulfone was rapid, > 50% of the administered compound dissipating within 7 days after application. Peak concentrations of the aldicarb sulfoxide (8.24 mg/kg) and aldicarb sulfone (0.8 mg/kg) were reached at day 14 after the application.

Ou et al. (1986) investigated the degradation and metabolism of ^{14}C-aldicarb in soils under aerobic and anaerobic conditions. They found that under aerobic conditions, aldicarb rapidly disappeared and aldicarb sulfoxide was rapidly formed; the latter in turn was slowly oxidized to aldicarb sulfone. The sulfoxide was the principal metabolite in soils under strictly aerobic conditions. Although the parent compound aldicarb persisted considerably longer in anaerobic soils, anaerobic half-lives for total toxic residue (aldicarb, aldicarb sulfoxide, and aldicarb sulfone) in subsurface soils were significantly shorter than under aerobic conditions.

A number of factors, including soil texture and type, soil organic content, soil moisture levels, time, and temperature, affect the rate of aldicarb degradations (Coppedge et al., 1967; Bull, 1968; Bull et al., 1970; Andrawes et al., 1971a; Suspak et al., 1977). Bull et al. (1970) reported that soil pH had no significant effect on the breakdown of aldicarb, but Supak et al. (1977) noted an increase in the rate of degradation when the pH was lowered.

Lightfoot & Thorne (1987) investigated the degradation of aldicarb, aldicarb sulfoxide, and aldicarb sulfone in the laboratory using distilled water, water extracted from soil, and water with soil particles (Table 3). Degradation

Table 3. Degradation rates for aldicarb, aldicarb sulfoxide, and aldicarb sulfone[a]

	Half-life at 25 °C (days)[b]	
	Aldicarb	Total carbamates[c]
Plough-layer soil		
sterilized	2.5 (2.3-2.6)	10 (7-16)
unsterilized	1.0 (0.9-1.1)	44 (39-50)
Soil water		
sterilized	1679 (1056-4064)	1924 (1133-6370)
unsterilized	156 (143-176)	175 (158-195)
Distilled water (no buffers)	671 (507-994)	697 (518-1064)
Saturated zone soil and water		
sterilized	15 (14-16)	16 (15-18)
unsterilized	37 (33-42)	123 (115-132)

[a] From: Lightfoot & Thorne (1987).
[b] Values in parentheses represent 95% confidence intervals.
[c] Aldicarb, aldicarb sulfoxide, and aldicarb sulfone.
  pH measurements
   sterilized soil water: 6.6-7.0 for 238 days; 4.8-5.0 at day 368
   unsterilized soil water: 6.6-6.7 for 56 days; 4.2-4.4 at day 238, 3.2 at day 368
   distilled water: 7.3-7.5 for 238 days, 6.2-6.8 at day 368
   saturated zone soil and water: 4.1-4.5 throughout entire study.

of all three compounds was greatest in the uppermost "plough" layer of the soil profile and much higher in the presence of soil particulates. Even after sterilization of the soil, degradation was fast in this layer, indicating that the effect of particulate matter is not entirely microbial. Degradation continued in the saturated zone (ground water) at a slower rate (particularly for the sulfoxide and sulfone). A further series of experiments investigated the degradation of mixtures of aldicarb sulfoxide and sulfone in soil and water from the saturated zone of two soil types (Table 4). The half-life was longer in the acidic Harrellsville soil than the alkaline Livingston soil. As in the case of laboratory experiments, the presence of particulates considerably increased the rate of degradation of the carbamates. Investigation of many variables in the laboratory led the authors to conclude that pH, temperature, redox potential, and perhaps the presence of trace substances can all affect degradation rates. They believed that laboratory experimentation could not provide definitive results without the

Table 4. Degradation rates for aldicarb sulfoxide and aldicarb sulfone mixtures in groundwater degradation mechanism studies[a]

Soil type and medium	Sterilized (25 °C)		Unsterilized (25 °C)	
	Half-life[b]	pH[c]	Half-life[b]	pH[c]
Harrellsville, NC				
saturated zone soil and water			137 (117-165)	5
Harrellsville, NC (first set)				
saturated zone soil and water	378 (287-550)	4.3	1910 (1170-5180)	4.2
coarse-filtered water	1100 (760-1970)	4.6	> 2000	4.6
fine-filtered water	> 2000	4.6	> 2000	4.2
Livingston, CA (original data)				
saturated zone soil and water			8 (7-10)	7
Livingston, CA				
saturated zone soil and water	1.3 (1.2-1.4)	9.0	7.5 (6.9-8.1)	8.4
coarse-filtered water	19 (17-22)	7.7	6.0 (5.7-6.3)	8.3

[a] From: Lightfoot & Thorne (1987).
[b] Half-life (days) for carbamate residues. Values in parentheses represent 95% confidence intervals. Since the experiments were conducted for only 1 year, half-life estimates greater than about 600 days are not as reliable as other estimates. Half-lives longer than about 2000 days could not be determined.
[c] Approximate average value during experiment.

identification of critical variables and that field observation was a more reliable indicator of aldicarb degradation

Coppedge et al. (1977) studied the movement and persistence of aldicarb in four different types of soil in laboratory and field settings using a radiolabelled substrate. Samples of clay, loam, "muck" (soil with high organic content), and sand were packed in polypropylene columns (63 x 128 mm), saturated with water, and maintained at 25 °C throughout the study. Radiolabelled aldicarb granules (34 mg) were applied to each column at a point 38 mm below the soil surface. Water was then applied to each soil column at a rate of 2.5 cm/week for the next 7 weeks. The water eluted through the columns was collected and analysed for radiolabel. At the end of the 7-week period, the soil was removed in layers 25 mm thick and analysed for residual radiolabel. The results of this study are shown in Tables 5 and 6. The radiolabel (< 1%) in the loam and clay soils remained in the upper layers of the column, close to where it had been applied. In the sand, the residual radiolabel (2-3%) passed through to the lower parts of the column. A much higher percentage (5-6%) of the radiolabel was retained in the muck soil column and was evenly distributed along the column. The radiolabel leached into the water eluted from the sand was 8-10 times greater than that from the other soil types. The nature of the decomposition products (ultimately shown to be carbon dioxide) resulted in some loss to the atmosphere surrounding the soils. The data in Table 6 indicate that most of the radioactivity retained in clay and loam soils represented aldicarb, sulfoxide whereas that in sand largely represented the parent compound. Greater leaching through sand decreased loss to the atmosphere by degradation to carbon dioxide.

Coppedge et al. (1977) also studied the persistence of aldicarb using field lysimeters. Aldicarb (34 mg), labelled with ^{35}S, was added to columns (63 x 128 mm) containing Lufkin fine sandy loam soil at a point 76 mm below the surface. The contents were moistened with water and then buried in the same type of soil at a depth where the insecticide granules were 152 mm below the surface. The experiment lasted for 7 weeks and rain was the only other source of moisture. The column recovered 3 days

Table 5. Distribution and persistence of ^{14}C-aldicarb equivalents in soil columns[a,b]

Soil type	Percentage of total dose in the various layers						Total extracted from soil	Unextractable residue from soil	Percentage of total dose		
	0-25[c]	25-50	50-75	75-100	100-128				In leached water[d]	Recovered	Lost
Houston clay	0.4	0.1	0.1	T	T		0.6	2.5	12.5	15.6	84.4
Lufkin loam	1.2	0.3	0.1	0.1	T		1.7	3.0	3.9	8.6	91.4
Coarse sand	T	T	0.2	0.5	2.0		2.7	0.2	84.0	86.9	13.1
Muck	8.7	5.3	8.5	5.6	4.8		32.9	7.1	3.5	43.5	56.5

[a] From: Coppedge et al. (1977).
[b] Results are the average from triplicate samples. Trace amounts (T) = < 0.1% of total dose.
[c] Layers are indicated by the distance (in mm) from the surface.
[d] Water that passed through the columns after the weekly addition of moisture.

Table 6. ^{14}C-labelled aldicarb and metabolites in water eluted through soil columns[a,b]

Soil type and compounds	Percentage of total dose recovered at indicated days after treatment								
	3	10	16	23	29	35	41	47	53
Clay									
aldicarb			0.5	0.2		T	0		
sulfoxide			3.2	1.9		0.4	0.2		
sulfone			0	T		T	0		
other metabolites			0.7	0.6		0.3	0.2		
Total	0	3.2	**4.4**	**2.7**	**0.8**	**0.7**	**0.4**	**0.3**	**0**
Accumulative total	0	3.2	**7.6**	**10.3**	**11.1**	**11.8**	**12.2**	**12.5**	**12.5**
Sand									
aldicarb			7.3	31.5		5.0	5.4	2.3	
sulfoxide			0.9	2.6		1.6	2.0	2.1	
sulfone			0	0		0	0	0	
other metabolites			0.2	1.9		0.4	0.5	1.1	
Total	0	3.5	**8.4**	**36.0**	**9.2**	**7.0**	**7.9**	**5.5**	**6.7**
Accumulative total	0	3.5	**11.9**	**47.9**	**57.1**	**64.1**	**72.0**	**77.5**	**84.0**

Table 6 (contd).

Loam									
aldicarb				T	T		T	0	
sulfoxide	0.7	0.7	0.9	0.3	0.2	0.3	0.2	0.3	0.3
sulfone			0	0		T	T		
other metabolites			0.2	T	0.2	T	0.1	0.2	
Total	0	0	1.1	0.3	0.4	0.3	0.3	0.5	0.3
Accumulative total	0	0.7	1.8	2.1	2.5	2.8	3.1	3.6	3.9
Muck									
aldicarb					T				
sulfoxide					0.1				
sulfone					0				
other metabolites					0.2				
Total	0	0.2	0.6	0.9	0.9	0.3	0.1	0.3	0.3
Accumulative total	0	0.2	0.8	1.7	2.6	2.9	3.0	3.3	3.6

[a] From: Coppedge et al. (1977).
[b] Results are the average from triplicate samples. Trace amounts (T) = < 0.1% of total dose. Where a "total" value is given without values for each component, the volume of samples was insufficient for individual analyses.

after the application yielded 71% of the radiolabel, while the column recovered at the end of 7 weeks yielded only 0.9%. This suggested an approximate half-life for the aldicarb of < 1 week, and the label distribution suggested an upward movement through volatilization of the decomposition products. The authors therefore concluded that there was little danger that aldicarb would move into the underground water supply in this type of soil.

Bowman (1988) studied the mobility and persistence of aldicarb using field lysimeters containing cores (diameter, 15 cm; length, 70 cm) of Plainfield sand. Half of the cores received only rainfall, while the remainder received rainfall plus simulated rainfall (50.8 mm) on the second and eighth days after treatment, followed by simulated irrigation for the duration of the study. The results of this study indicated that under normal rainfall about 9% of the applied aldicarb leached out of the soil cores as sulfoxide or sulfone, whereas, in cores receiving supplementary watering, up to 64% of applied aldicarb appeared in the effluent principally as sulfoxide or sulfone.

Andrawes et al. (1971a) studied the fate of radiolabelled aldicarb (S-methyl-^{14}C-Temik) in potato fields. The initial soil concentration was 13.1 mg/kg, which fell to 25.6 and 9.5% of the applied amount after 7 and 90 days, respectively. Samples taken as early as 30 min after the application showed that 12.7% of the aldicarb had already been converted to aldicarb sufoxide. By day 7 it had increased to 48%. In fallow soil, aldicarb was applied as an acetone/water solution at the same level as that used in the planted field. The dissipation of ^{14}C residues occurred at a relatively slow rate for the first 2 weeks and then at a faster rate. The breakdown products in both the fallow and planted fields were essentially the same.

LaFrance et al. (1988) studied the adsorption characteristics of aldicarb on loamy sand and its mobility through a water-saturated column in the presence of dissolved organic matter. The results of these studies suggested that aldicarb does not undergo appreciable complexation with dissolved humic materials found in the interstitial water of the unsaturated zones. Thus the presence of dissolved humic substances in the soil interstitial water should not markedly affect the transport of the pesticide towards the water table.

Woodham et al. (1973a) studied the lateral movement of aldicarb in sandy loam soil. They applied the granular commercial formulation of the pesticide (Temik 10G) to irrigated and non-irrigated fields at a rate of 16.8 kg/ha and placed it 15-20 cm to the side of cotton seedlings and 12.5-15 cm deep. Soil samples were collected throughout the growing season from a depth of 15 cm, from the bottom of a creek adjacent to a treated field, and from sites 0.40 and 1.61 km downstream. The aldicarb used in this study was found to have a short residence time. Levels in the treated field fell to 15% within one month. Only 8% remained after 47 days. No residues were found after 4 months and no aldicarb was detected either between rows or in the bed of the creek that collected water drainage. The authors concluded that aldicarb was translocated into crop plants and weeds but that there would be no carry-over of aldicarb or its metabolites from one growing season to another (Woodham et al., 1973b). The results of studies by Andrawes et al. (1971a) and Maitlen & Powell (1982) agree with the observations of Woodham and his colleagues. Gonzalez & Weaver (1986) failed to detect aldicarb or its breakdown products in run-off water from a field treated with aldicarb in California, USA.

The method and timing of application can also affect the migration and degradation of aldicarb (Jones et al., 1986). Aldicarb was applied in-furrow during the planting of potatoes and as a top-dressing at crop emergence. At the end of the growing season the residues from the first application were found primarily in the top 0.6 m of soil, and the residues from the emergence application were found primarily in the top 0.3 m of soil.

In a three-year Wisconsin potato field study (sandy plain), Fathulla et al. (1988) monitored aldicarb residues in the saturated zone ground water under fluctuating conditions of temperature, pH, and total hardness. Soils were well drained sands, loamy sands or sandy loams (with 1 to 2% organic matter). The water table was high with a depth to the saturated zone of between 1.3 and 4.6 m. Sampling wells were bored to a maximum of 7.5 m for groundwater sampling. Rothschild et al. (1982) had found all residues of aldicarb (and its breakdown products) within the upper 1.5 m of the ground water in the same area in an earlier study. This is consistent with the views of both groups of authors that movement of aldicarb will occur in these aquifers. The report of Fathulla et al. (1988) indicated that detection and persistence of aldicarb in the ground water were dependent on alkalinity and temperature. Movement of aldicarb was lateral as well as vertical and the authors emphasized the importance of seasonal changes in water table depth and precipitation as factors influencing movement. Degradation by microorganisms in the upper layers of the soil and ground water was noted and identified as a major factor in the short-term fate of the aldicarb. Hegg et al. (1988) measured the movement and degradation of aldicarb in a loamy sand soil in South Carolina, USA, and found that it degraded at a rate corresponding to a half-life of 9 days with essentially no residues present 4 months after application. This was a faster loss of aldicarb from the soil than in comparable studies in neighbouring areas. Using the unsaturated plant root zone model (PRZM) with rainfall records from 15 years, aldicarb residues were predicted to be limited to the upper 1.5 m, regardless of year-to-year variations in rainfall.

Pacenka et al. (1987) sampled both soil cores and ground water from sites on Long Island (New York, USA), where earlier surveys had suggested contamination of wells with aldicarb and its breakdown products (the sulfone and sulfoxide). Three study areas were chosen with shallow (3 m), medium (10 m), and deep (30 m) water tables. All were overlain with sandy soils. Soil cores, driven to the depth of the water table, were taken from a field where aldicarb had been applied to potatoes and from surrounding areas. Ground water was sampled from 188 wells of varying depth and at different distances from the aldicarb source. Results indicated that the residence time of aldicarb (including the sulfone and sulfoxide) in the soil depended on the depth of the water table and, hence, the overlying unsaturated zone. In the shallow and medium depth water table sites, all aldicarb residues had disappeared within 3 years of the last use of the compound. In deeper unsaturated layers, aldicarb residues were present at increasing concentrations in soil water from 10 m down to the water table at 30 m. The uppermost 10 m was free of residues. Analysis of the groundwater samples showed lateral movement of residues extending from 120 m to 270 m "downstream" of the source in a single year. It was calculated that the relatively shallow aquifer in the area (which lay over a deeper aquifer capped by an impervious layer of clay) would flush residues from the area completely within 100 years and lead to concentrations below the drinking-water guideline level (New York) of 7 µg/litre being attained between 1987 and 2010 (depending on assumptions for dispersion and degradation). Pacenka et al. (1987) revised this figure downwards on the basis of their more extensive field observations, although no firm figure could be advanced.

Studies in other geographical areas of the USA, including those showing some residues of aldicarb or the sulfoxide and sulfone in wells, have demonstrated a shorter residence time and more rapid degradation than in the Long Island study (Jones et al., 1986; Wyman et al., 1987; Jones, 1986, 1987). In these studies there was little lateral movement of the ground water in the saturated zone. Water table levels in these areas were generally high and much of the sampling of the ground water was in the top 4-5 m of the saturated zone. Much greater lateral movement of ground water in the Florida Ridge area at a shallower depth than similar movement in Long Island also shifted the aldicarb residues away from the treated area. However, degradation was sufficiently fast in these soils to reduce the chance of contamination of wells used for drinking-water. An impervious layer 6 m down would prevent deeper contamination in this area (Jones et al., 1987a).

A review of well and groundwater monitoring of aldicarb residues throughout the USA has been published by Lorber et al. (1989, 1990), which indicates geographical areas at greatest risk of water contamination and local restrictions on the use of aldicarb.

4.1.3 Vegetation and wildlife

The uptake of aldicarb and its residues by food crops and plants has been reported in several studies (Andrawes et al., 1974; Maitlen & Powell, 1982). Residue levels in plants and crops grown in aldicarb-treated soil are given in Table 7. Of the many varieties and species of birds and mammals studied, only the oriole had aldicarb residues (0.07 mg aldicarb equivalents per kg) in its tissues (Woodham et al., 1973b).

In a study by Iwata et al. (1977), aldicarb was applied to the soil in orange groves at rates of 2.8, 5.6, 11.2, and 22.4 kg ai/ha. Residues found on day 118 after application in the soil were 0.03, 0.16, 0.20, and 0.42 mg/kg, respectively. On day 193, samples were taken from the pulp of oranges grown in soil that had been given the highest amount (22.4 kg ai/ha) of aldicarb. The residues in these samples ranged from 0.02-0.03 mg/kg.

After aldicarb was applied to the leaves of young cotton plants under field conditions, it was not translocated to other parts of the plant to any great extent (Bull, 1968). Two weeks after application, 93% of the recovered radiolabel was found at the application site. The remainder was spread evenly throughout the plant, including the roots and fruit.

4.2 Biotransformation

In plants, aldicarb is metabolized by processes involving oxidation to the sulfoxide and sulfone, as well as by hydrolysis to the corresponding oximes and, ultimately, to the nitrile.

There have been several studies on the metabolism of aldicarb by the cotton plant. Metcalf et al. (1966) found that aldicarb was completely converted within 4-9 days to the sulfoxide, which was then hydrolysed to the oxime. The subsequent oxidation of the sulfoxide to the sulfone occurred more slowly and was found to lead to bioaccumulation in aged residues (Coppedge et al., 1967).

When aldicarb (10 µl of an aqueous solution containing 10 µg aldicarb) was applied to the leaves of cotton plants, 7.1% of the administered dose was converted to the sulfoxide within 15 min. Two days later there was no residual aldicarb in or on the plant tissues, and the principal metabolite (78.4% of the initial dose) was the sulfoxide. After 8 days, 7.4% of the initial dose was found as

Table 7. Residues (in mg/kg) of aldicarb and its sulfoxide and sulfone metabolites found in various crops grown in aldicarb-treated soil[a,b]

Replicate no.	Potato leaves[c] (70)[d]	Potato leaves (408)	Alfalfa (transplanted) (456)	Alfalfa (seeded) (456)	Mint foliage (408)	Mustard greens (408)	Radish tops (408)	Radish roots (408)
3.4 kg a/ha application								
1	7.65	0.52	0.14	0.16	0.02	ND	0.08	ND
2	7.93	0.15	ND	0.04	0.01	0.03	0.07	ND
3	8.11	1.34	0.09	0.05	0.05	0.08	0.05	ND
4	8.74	1.27	0.24	0.14	0.10			
5	9.60	1.03	0.13	0.24	0.06			
Average	8.41	0.66	0.12	0.13	0.05	0.04	0.07	ND
15.0 kg a/ha application								
1	19.30	0.69	0.89	0.89	0.64	ND	0.27	0.04
2	14.90	1.10	0.34	1.47	0.92	0.26	0.27	0.05
3	20.80	1.12	0.43	0.26	0.37	0.40	0.18	0.03
4	19.40	0.50	0.76	0.61	0.23			
5	22.60	1.96	1.37	8.37	1.55			
Average	19.40	1.07	0.76	2.32	0.74	0.22	0.24	0.04

[a] From: Maitlen & Powell (1982).
[b] Residues in this table were determined by oxidizing the aldicarb, aldicarb sulfoxide, and aldicarb sulfone and then determining them as one combined compound, aldicarb sulfone. ND = none detected; the lower limit of reliable detection for these samples was < 5.0 ng/aliquot analysed or < 0.02 mg/kg.
[c] These samples are from the crop of 1979. All others are from the crop of 1980.
[d] Figures in parentheses are the interval in days between treatment of soil and sampling of plants.

the sulfone while the nitrile sulfoxide and an unidentified metabolite were the final products of decomposition (Bull, 1968).

4.3 Interaction with other physical, chemical or biological factors

4.3.1 Soil microorganisms

Kuseske et al. (1974) studied the degradation of aldicarb under aerobic and anaerobic conditions and found that degradation was much slower under anaerobic conditions. Jones (1976) studied the metabolism of aldicarb by five common soil fungi. The potential for aldicarb detoxification by these fungi (in decreasing order) was as follows: *Gliocladium catenulatum* > *Penicillium multicolor* = *Cunninghamella elegans* > *Rhizoctonia* sp. > *Trichoderma harzianum*. The major organosoluble metabolites were identified as aldicarb sulfoxide, the oxime sulfoxide, the nitrile sulfoxide, and smaller amounts of the corresponding sulfones, indicating that the metabolic pathways were similar to those found in higher plants and animals.

Spurr & Sousa (1966, 1974) tested the effects of aldicarb and its metabolites on pathogenic and saprophytic microorganisms and found that some of the microorganisms appeared to use aldicarb as a carbon source. The various bacteria and fungi used in these tests showed no growth inhibition when aldicarb was added at levels up to 20 times those usually used in field conditions.

5. ENVIRONMENTAL LEVELS AND HUMAN EXPOSURE

5.1 Environmental levels

5.1.1 Air

Since aldicarb is applied in granular form to the soil surface, it reaches the atmosphere only by upward migration and by volatilization. Thus, it is not transported to the atmosphere to any great extent and so is not expected to contribute a significant health threat from this source. In a volatilization study (Supak et al., 1977), a special apparatus was designed to determine the volatility of aldicarb from the soil. The air eluted from the apparatus after it had passed over soil samples containing dispersed aldicarb was analysed by the method of Maitlen et al. (1970). This method allowed the quantitative analysis of aldicarb and its two oxidation products, the sulfoxide and sulfone, both of which are toxic. Nontoxic decomposition products, such as the sulfoxide and sulfone oximes, both of which interfere with the determination of aldicarb sulfone by this method, were removed by LC. When aldicarb was mixed with soil to a concentration of 1 mg/kg, only 2 µg of aldicarb volatilized over the first 9 days of the experiment and subsequent losses increased to a steady-state rate of approximately 1 µg/day. According to the authors, this rate of volatilization was almost negligible and not high enough to cause a potential health hazard.

5.1.2 Water

Run-off to surface water and leaching to aquifers used as sources of water for human consumption have been investigated. Aldicarb residues have been found in drinking-water wells in New York (Wilkinson et al., 1983; Varma et al., 1983), Wisconsin (Rothschild et al., 1982), and Florida (Miller et al., 1985). The US EPA groundwater team reported that they had found groundwater residues in 22 states (US EPA, 1988b). In Canada, water samples taken from private wells showed contamination with aldicarb up to 6.0 µg/litre; ground water from Quebec (maximum of 28 µg/litre) and Ontario (maximum of 1.1 µg/litre) also contained detectable levels (Hiebsch, 1988).

Prince Edward Island, Canada, is wholly dependent upon ground water from a highly permeable sandstone aquifer for domestic, agricultural, and industrial use. Priddle et al. (1989) reported that 12% of monitored wells exceeded the Canadian drinking-water guideline of 9 µg/litre for aldicarb. The maximum level detected was 15 µg/litre.

Following extensive agricultural use of aldicarb and as a result of a combination of environmental and hydrological conditions on eastern Long Island, New York, in 1978 the insecticide and its metabolites had leached into groundwater aquifers that constitute the major source of drinking-water for local inhabitants. In December 1978, detectable levels of aldicarb were found in 20 of 31 water sources; similar results were obtained in the following June. When both private and community wells located near potato farms were sampled in August 1979, analyses revealed detectable levels of aldicarb in potable water. In March 1980, the Department of Health Services in Suffolk County, New York, undertook an extensive sampling programme that included nearly 8000 wells. Union Carbide performed the analyses, with the New York Department of Health serving as the quality control arm. Levels of aldicarb ranging from trace amounts to > 400 µg/litre were detected in 27% of the wells sampled. Baier & Moran (1981) reported that of 7802 wells sampled, 5745 (73.6%) did not have detectable concentrations of aldicarb, 1025 (13.1%) had concentrations in excess of the 7 µg/litre guideline of the New York State Department of Health, and the remaining 1032 (13.3%) had trace amounts of this insecticide.

Aldicarb has been found at levels of 1-50 µg/litre in the ground water of the USA (Cohen et al., 1986; de Hann, 1988).

The contamination of the Long Island (New York) aquifer by aldicarb at levels of up to 500 µg/litre (in one well) was attributed by Marshall (1985) to a combination of circumstances (high rainfall, coarse sandy soil, low soil temperatures, and a shallow water table) that favoured leaching. There have been some predictions that this undesirable situation would persist for only a year or two, but also some suggestions that wells could remain contaminated for up to a century. Marshall (1985) also voiced concern that under anaerobic conditions in cool climates, such as those in northern regions, the breakdown of aldicarb and its residues would be a much slower process. Contamination would also be favoured by heavy usage of Temik.

During 1982, aldicarb was identified in several wells in the state of Florida (Miller et al., 1985). The state Commission of Agriculture and Consumer Services subsequently banned the use of Temik on citrus crops in 1983. A University of Florida task force was appointed to sample the 10 largest drinking-water systems that obtained water from groundwater sources in 35 counties. Neither aldicarb nor its oxidative sulfoxide or sulfone metabolites were detected in any of the almost 400 samples collected.

During the application season of 1984 (January to April), 2040 tonnes of aldicarb was used on citrus fruits at a rate of 5.6 kg ai/ha in more than 30 counties in Florida. No residues were detected in samples taken from community water systems, but trace amounts of aldicarb, aldicarb sulfoxide, and aldicarb sulfone were found in the Calloosahatchee River from which Lee County draws its drinking-water. (However, no residues were found in finished drinking-water in Lee County). The authors stated that the persistence of aldicarb and its metabolites in shallow ground water may also contaminate drinking-water. The results of a monitoring study by the Union Carbide Corporation (UCC) showed that in shallow ground water aldicarb can move further from its application point than originally predicted.

5.1.3 Food and feed

Residues have been detected on a variety of crops for which aldicarb is used (see section 3.2.1). In the USA, aldicarb intoxication from eating contaminated watermelons has been reported in California (Jackson et al., 1986) and in Oregon (Green et al., 1987), and two episodes of poisoning from eating aldicarb-contaminated cucumbers have been reported in Nebraska (Goes et al., 1980). Store-bought cucumbers, grown hydroponically, were found to contain between 7 and 10 mg aldicarb/kg (Aaronson et al., 1980). It should be noted that aldicarb is not approved for use on these crops.

Laski & Vannelli (1984) reported the results of a survey of potatoes grown in New York State in 1982. Fifty samples, each consisting of 9 kg, were collected after harvest from four areas. In each of these areas, except one (Long Island), aldicarb was applied at rates of 14 to 22 kg/ha at planting stage. Samples were analysed for aldicarb, aldicarb sulfoxide, and aldicarb sulfone by the method of Krause (1980). Over 50% (23 out of 43) of potato samples obtained from areas where aldicarb was applied were positive for aldicarb sulfoxide (trace to 0.48 mg/kg) and/or sulfone (trace to 0.20 mg/kg), but aldicarb itself was not detected. No residues were found in any of the 7 samples from Long Island. The maximum concentrations were detected in samples from the North Eastern location, where there is sandy soil. Potatoes with the maximum concentration (0.48 mg/kg) were found to contain two and a half times higher concentrations (1.2 mg/kg) when reanalysed by a more sensitive method (Union Carbide, 1983). The investigators suggested that soil type and climatic conditions influenced residues in the crops.

When Krause (1985b) analysed aldicarb and its oxidative metabolites in "market basket" potatoes, he detected levels of aldicarb sulfone ranging from < 0.01 to 0.18 mg/kg and of aldicarb sulfoxide from < 0.01 to 0.61 mg/kg. All 39 samples collected between 1980 and 1983 contained residues of aldicarb or its metabolites.

Potato samples collected from farms in the north-central part of New York, where soil is of the wet muck type, contained lower aldicarb residues than did the rocky-sandy soil type found in the north-eastern part of the state, even though application rates were the same in both areas. These lower residue levels were the result of aldicarb decomposition associated with moisture. Cairns et al. (1984) described the persistence of aldicarb in fresh potatoes.

Peterson & Gregorio (1988) reported upper 95 percentile residue levels of 0.0677 mg/kg in raw potatoes (tolerance = 1 mg/kg), 0.0658 mg/kg in fresh bananas (tolerance = 0.3 mg/kg), and 0.0212 mg/kg in grapefruit (tolerance = 0.3 mg/kg) in a market basket survey conducted in the USA (national food survey). These authors also reported a maximum residue level of 0.82 mg/kg in raw potatoes obtained in controlled field trials, as well as upper 95 percentile residue levels as high as 0.43 mg/kg in raw potatoes, 0.12 mg/kg in bananas, and 0.17 mg/kg in citrus products, estimated from the distribution of residue levels obtained in field trials.

5.2 General population exposure

The general population may be exposed to aldicarb and its residues primarily through the ingestion of food containing aldicarb and from contaminated water, as discussed in sections 5.1.2, 5.1.3., and section 8. The largest documented episode of foodborne pesticide poisoning in North American history occurred in July 1985. This resulted from the consumption of Californian water-melons contaminated with up to 3.3 mg/kg of aldicarb sulfoxide (Ting & Kho, 1986).

Hirsch et al. (1987) reported 140 cases of poisoning incidences in the Vancouver area of British Columbia, Canada. A review of the onset of symptoms and food consumed suggested illness associated with eating cucumbers contaminated with aldicarb. Analytical investigations confirmed that the cucumbers from one producer contained residues of total aldicarb up to 26 mg/kg.

Petersen & Gregorio (1988) reported the results of a comprehensive analysis of aldicarb data from controlled field residue studies and provided estimates of the upper 95 percentile of residues in foods in the USA. The analysis showed that daily exposure at the upper 95 percentile consumption rate for aldicarb-treated commodities containing the estimated upper 95 percentile aldicarb residue levels would be approximately one-quarter of the daily exposure calculated by assuming that all of the aldicarb-treated commodities contained residues at the tolerance levels (e.g., 1.77 µg/kg per day versus 6.38 µg/kg per day for the USA population). In addition, Petersen & Gregorio (1988) presented the results of a statistically designed national food survey on the five commodities that were estimated to be responsible for more than 90% of the dietary exposure to aldicarb residues in the USA (bananas, white potatoes, sweet potatoes, oranges, and grapefruit). Daily exposure to aldicarb at the 95 percentile consumption rate for aldicarb-treated commodities containing the

95 percentile aldicarb residue levels, as estimated from the national food survey, would be approximately 6% of the daily exposure calculated by assuming aldicarb residue levels at the tolerance levels (e.g. 0.40 µg/kg body weight per day versus 6.38 µg/kg per day for the USA population).

The highest daily exposure estimated from the results of the national food survey was 0.89 µg/kg per day for non-nursing infants and children (1-6 years of age).

A US EPA survey indicated that the vast majority of wells contained levels of aldicarb residues less than 10 µg/litre and noted that heat treatment of water used in cooking would result in aldicarb residues no higher than 5 µg/litre (Cohen et al., 1986).

Accidental leaks of several gases at a plant producing aldicarb in Institute, West Virginia, USA, required 135 people to be the hospitalized (Marshall, 1985).

5.3 Occupational exposure during manufacture, formulation or use

The dangers of inadequate safety precautions and improper dress and handling procedures are discussed in section 8. People involved in the manufacture and field application of aldicarb are potentially at higher risk than the general population (Doull et al., 1980) and should always take proper safety precautions.

6. KINETICS AND METABOLISM

6.1 Absorption

A number of studies on various mammalian and non-mammalian species have shown that aldicarb, as well as its sulfoxide and sulfone metabolites, is absorbed readily and almost completely from the gastrointestinal tract (Knaak et al., 1966a,b; Andrawes et al., 1967; Dorough & Ivie, 1968; Dorough et al., 1970; Hicks et al., 1972; Cambon et al., 1979). Andrawes et al. (1967) reported that the uptake of aldicarb and aldicarb sulfoxide from the gastrointestinal tract of the rat was rapid and efficient. They recovered 80-90% of the radiolabel in the urine during the first 24 h after administration. Their observation was substantiated by Knaak et al. (1966a,b), who also recovered > 90% of the administered oral dose in rats.

Cambon et al. (1979) reported the rapid uptake of aldicarb in pregnant rats. The rats showed overt signs of depression of cholinesterase activity < 5 min after they were given single oral doses of aldicarb ranging from 0.001 to 0.10 mg/kg. At all dose levels, acetylcholinesterase activity was significantly decreased in fetal blood, brain, and liver 1 h after dosing.

Dorough et al. (1970) recovered 92% of the doses (0.006-0.52 mg/kg per day) of aldicarb and aldicarb sulfone in the urine of lactating Holstein cows dosed during a 14-day period. Dorough & Ivie (1968) found that > 90% of a single dose of 0.1 mg/kg administered orally to lactating Jersey cows was absorbed and excreted in the urine. In laying hens, oral doses of aldicarb and aldicarb sulfone were administered in a 21-day short-term feeding study and in a single capsule dose study, respectively. In the short-term feeding study, 80-85% of each daily dose was excreted in the faeces during the following 24 h, while 90% of the total dose consumed was excreted within one week after the cessation of aldicarb intake. In the single dose study, 90% of the single oral dose was excreted within 10 days (Hicks et al., 1972).

Feldman & Maibach (1970) reported the relatively efficient dermal uptake of carbamate insecticides in man

(73.9% of a dermally applied dose of carbaryl was absorbed over a period of 5 days compared with 10% for five other representative pesticides). The percutaneous uptake of aldicarb in water or in toluene has also been demonstrated qualitatively in rabbits (Kuhr & Dorough, 1976; Martin & Worthing, 1977) and in rats (Gaines, 1969).

6.2 Distribution

The rapid depression of acetylcholinesterase activity in fetal and maternal blood and tissues observed after the oral administration of aldicarb to pregnant rats demonstrated that aldicarb or its toxic metabolites (the sulfoxide and sulfone) are distributed to the tissues by the systemic circulation (Cambon et al., 1979, 1980). The quantitative distribution of radiolabelled aldicarb and its metabolites in the tissues of female rats, given a single oral dose of 0.4 mg aldicarb/kg, is shown in Table 8 (Andrawes et al., 1967). Aldicarb and its residues appeared to be distributed among the various tissues examined with no tendency to be sequestered or accumulated in any one tissue, since animals killed from 5 to 11 days after dosing had no detectable radiolabelled residues.

Aldicarb and its metabolites were found to be concentrated in the livers of cows fed 0.12, 0.6, or 1.2 mg aldicarb/kg diet for up to 14 days (Dorough et al., 1970). Levels of the radiolabel in muscle, fat, and bone were low or below the detection levels. In a previous study, Dorough & Ivie (1968) found that 3% of the radiolabel was excreted in the milk of a lactating cow after a single oral dose of 0.1 mg/kg.

Hicks et al. (1972) conducted a study in which single oral doses (0.7 mg/kg) of aldicarb or a 1:1 molar ratio of aldicarb and aldicarb sulfone were administered to laying hens. The radiolabel equivalents were greatest in the liver and kidneys for the first 24 h, much lower levels being found in fat and muscle. In a second study, aldicarb/aldicarb sulfone was administered at 0.1, 1.0, or 20 mg/kg diet for 21 days. Distribution to the tissues after this multiple dosing regimen was similar to that after the single dose, the highest residue levels appearing in the liver and kidneys.

Table 8. Total aldicarb equivalents (mg/kg) in tissues of rats treated orally with ^{35}S-aldicarb[a]

	Time period (days after dosing)[b]							
	Day 1		Day 2		Day 3		Day 4	
	W	D	W	D	W	D	W	D
Heart	0.12	0.44	0.09	0.32	0.08	0.29	0.11	0.38
Kidneys	0.16	0.56	0.08	0.25	0.06	0.16	0.07	0.21
Brain	0.11	0.35	0.02	0.08	0.08	0.25	0.05	0.19
Lungs	0.15	0.60	0.02	0.48	0.04	0.14	0.06	1.19
Spleen	0.27	1.08	0.04	0.12	0.10	0.37	0.05	0.17
Liver	0.16	0.28	0.07	0.22	0.07	0.21	0.05	0.14
Leg muscle	0.16	0.61	0.02	0.07	0.05	0.20	0.04	0.12
Fat	0.23	0.72	0.11	0.12	0.09	0.11	0.03	0.04
Bone	0.11	0.15	0.09	0.13	0.06	0.08	0.02	0.04
Stomach	0.19	0.64	0.07	0.26	0.08	0.29	0.06	0.19
Stomach contents	0.18	0.94	0.14	1.05	0.10	0.65	0.03	0.09
Small intestine	0.18	0.74	0.13	0.45	0.10	0.30	0.06	0.16
Small intestine contents	0.25	1.20	0.19	1.03	0.08	0.49	0.06	0.24
Large intestine	0.15	0.66	0.12	0.54	0.08	0.27	0.13	0.30
Large intestine contents	0.18	0.67	0.05	0.24	0.09	0.39	0.04	0.16
Blood	0.16	0.74	0.14	0.18	0.08	0.21	0.05	0.17

[a] From: Andrawes et al. (1967).
[b] W = wet weight; D = dry weight.

6.3 Metabolic transformation

Carbamates undergo a limited number of *in vivo* reactions: oxidation, reduction, hydrolysis, and conjugation (Ryan, 1971). In animals, the enzymes involved in these processes are found in the microsomal fraction of the liver homogenate. In the case of aldicarb, both oxidation of the sulfur to the sulfoxide and sulfone and hydrolysis of the carbamate ester group are involved (Andrawes et al., 1967). Although the hydrolysis reaction destroys insecticidal activity, both the sulfoxide and sulfone are active anticholinesterase agents (Andrawes et al., 1967; Bull et al., 1967; NAS, 1977). The metabolic pathways for aldicarb in the rat are shown in Fig. 1 (Wilkinson et al., 1983). The metabolism of aldicarb in animals usually results in the formation of the sulfoxide, sulfone, oxime sulfoxide, oxime sulfone, nitrile sulfoxide, nitrile sulfone, and at least five other metabolites (Knaak et al., 1966a,b; Dorough et al., 1970). Aldicarb metabolites formed by incubation with liver microsomal enzymes are similar to the metabolites formed in plants and insects (Oonnithan & Casida, 1967). The rapid conversion to the sulfoxide and sulfone has been demonstrated in plants (Metcalf et al., 1966; Coppedge et al., 1967) and animals (Andrawes et al., 1967; Dorough & Ivie, 1968).

In vitro studies by Oonnithan & Casida (1967) showed that the first stage in the metabolism of aldicarb involves the microsomal reduced nicotinamide adenine dinucleotide phosphate (NADPH) system to form the sulfoxide, but that the subsequent oxidation to the sulfone derivative occurs only to a small extent. Andrawes et al. (1967) confirmed these findings and showed that in the presence of the NADPH cofactor the production of metabolites increases by a factor of 15. The same authors also demonstrated that the principal urinary metabolites in the rat consist of hydrolytic products with only a small amount of carbamate. In studies with pig liver enzymes, Hajjar & Hodgson (1982) concluded that, under aerobic conditions and in the presence of NADPH, the FAD-dependent monooxygenase is responsible for the observed oxidation of the thio-ether in the primary metabolic step. The same authors found that sulfoxidation is enhanced rather than inhibited by *n*-octylamine, a known inhibitor of cytochrome P-450-dependent oxygenation.

6.4 Elimination and excretion in expired air, faeces, and urine

Most studies on the elimination and excretion of aldicarb and its metabolites have used the radiolabelled compound. No kinetic coefficients have been reported,

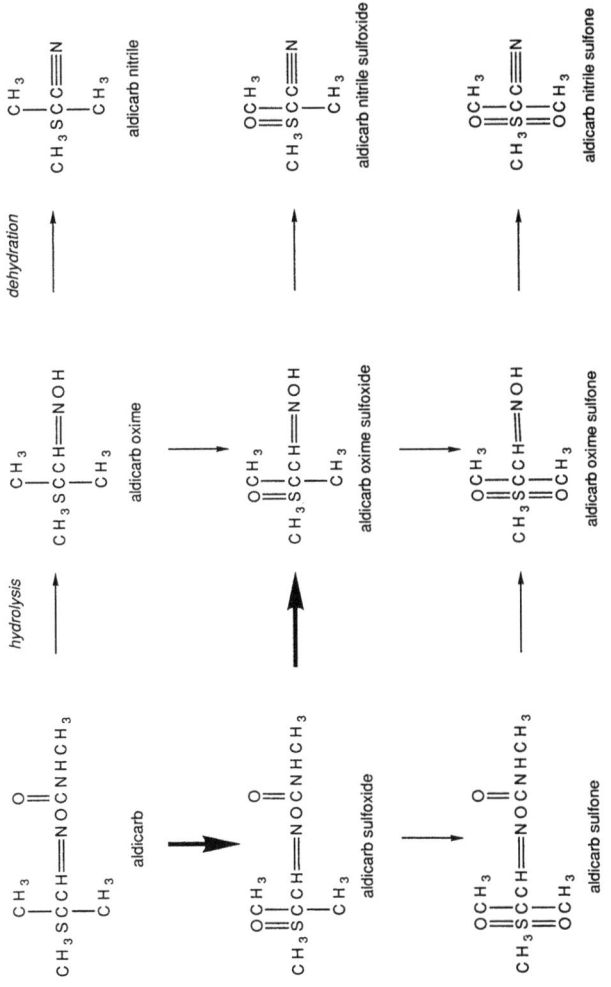

Fig. 1. Metabolism of aldicarb in rats. Modified from Wilkinson et al. (1983).

although studies in which rats (Knaak et al., 1966a,b; Andrawes et al., 1967; Dorough & Ivie, 1968; Marshall & Dorough, 1979), cows (Dorough & Ivie, 1968; Dorough et al., 1970), and chickens (Hicks et al., 1972) were used gave some information about the clearance rates, mechanisms, and routes of excretion. In all species, the principal excretion route for aldicarb and its metabolites (> 90%) is via the urine. A small amount of aldicarb and its metabolic products is excreted via the faeces (which is in part due to biliary excretion), or is exhaled as carbon dioxide.

The total excretion of S-methyl-C^{14}-, $tert$-butyl-C^{14}-, and N-methyl-C^{14}-labelled aldicarb by rats after oral dosing was investigated by Knaak et al. (1966a). Within 24 h, the total excretion of the S-methyl, $tert$-butyl, and N-methyl labels was approximately 90, 90, and 60%, respectively. For the S-methyl- and $tert$-butyl-labelled compounds, > 90% was excreted via the urine and only 1.1% of the radiolabel was excreted as carbon dioxide. In a study on rats dosed orally with aldicarb (labelled in a different position and with different radioisotopes), Andrawes et al. (1967) showed that > 80% of the applied dose (labelled with ^{14}C) was excreted over 24 days, while 6.6% was excreted in the faeces within 4 days.

The biliary excretion of aldicarb and its metabolites was studied by Marshall & Dorough (1979) in rats with cannulated bile ducts. A single oral dose of ^{14}C-thiomethyl aldicarb (0.1 mg/kg) in 0.2 ml of vegetable oil was given by intubation, and urine, bile, and faeces were collected over the next 72 h. Biliary excretion accounted for 2.6, 9.5, 22.9, 28.1, and 28.6% of the administered dose at 3, 6, 12, 24, and 48 h after dosing, respectively. More than 64% was excreted in the urine over the 48-h period, and < 1% was recovered from the faeces.

In a study by Dorough & Ivie (1968), 83% of an oral dose of 0.1 mg/kg given to a lactating cow was recovered in the urine within 24 h, this increasing to 90% over 22.5 days. Only 2.85% of the radiolabel was recovered in the faeces within 8 days after dosing. All samples of milk taken from 3 h to 22.5 days after dosing contained the radiolabel and accounted for 3.02% of the administered dose.

Hicks et al. (1972) dosed laying hens with ^{35}S-aldicarb or with a 1:1 molar ratio of ^{14}C-aldicarb and ^{14}C-aldicarb sulfone. The dose (0.7 mg/kg) was administered orally in a gelatin capsule. In both cases, the label was excreted rapidly; 75% of the radiolabel was recovered in the faeces within 24 h and > 80% was recovered within 48 h. Repeated dosing, twice a day for 21 days, resulted in a similar pattern of excretion, 80-85% of the daily dose being excreted in the faeces within 24 h after the administration of each dose.

7. EFFECTS ON LABORATORY MAMMALS AND *IN VITRO* TEST SYSTEMS

7.1 Single exposure

The acute oral and dermal toxicity of aldicarb has been studied in several species (Table 9). Oral LD_{50} values appear to be fairly consistent (0.3-0.9 mg/kg body weight in the rat) and not dependent on the carrier vehicle. Oral administration of the granular formulation of aldicarb gives LD_{50} values proportional to the active ingredient content (Carpenter & Smyth, 1965). The oral LD_{50} values for aldicarb sulfoxide and sulfone in rats are 0.88 mg/kg body weight and 25.0 mg/kg body weight, respectively (Weil, 1968). Dermal LD_{50} values vary with the mode of application and the carrier vehicle used. Several acute dermal toxicity studies using different carrier vehicles have been reported. The dermal 24-h LD_{50} in rabbits for a single application of aldicarb in water was 32 mg/kg body weight (West & Carpenter, 1966). However, when aldicarb was tested in propylene glycol, the observed dermal LD_{50} was 5 mg/kg body weight (Striegel & Carpenter, 1962). A dermal LD_{50} of 141 mg/kg body weight was reported in a 4-h exposure study on rabbits using dry Temik 10G formulation. On the basis of results of acute oral and dermal toxicity studies, aldicarb should be labelled as extremely hazardous (WHO, 1990b).

Carpenter & Smyth (1965) reported 100% mortality within 5 min when rats, mice, and guinea-pigs were exposed to aldicarb dust at a concentration of 200 mg/m^3. The rats and mice were more sensitive than the guinea-pigs. Rats survived a dust concentration of 6.7 mg/m^3 for 15 min, but five out of six died after 30 min. All rats survived for 8 h when exposed to a saturated vapour concentration. Rats were also less sensitive to aerosol concentrations than to similar concentrations of the dust. Two of six rats survived an 8-h exposure to an aerosol concentration of 7.6 mg/m^3. Weil & Carpenter (1970) determined an LD_{50} of 0.44 mg/kg body weight in rats by the intraperitoneal route.

Trutter (1989a) investigated the clinical effects and the effect on plasma cholinesterase and erythrocyte

Table 9. Acute toxicity of aldicarb and its formulation products

Compound	Route of administration	Vehicle	Species	LD$_{50}$ (mg/kg body weight)[a]	Reference
Technical aldicarb	oral		rat	0.93	Martin & Worthing (1977)
	oral	peanut oil	rat	M: 0.8 F: 0.65	Gaines (1969)
	oral	corn oil	rat	M: 0.09	Carpenter & Smyth (1965)
	oral	corn oil	rat	F: 1.0	Weiden et al. (1965)
	oral	not specified	mouse	0.3	Black et al. (1973)
	skin	xylene	rat	M: 3.0 F: 2.5	Gaines (1969)
	skin	not specified	rabbit	5.0	Weiden et al. (1965)
	skin	propylene glycol (5%)	rabbit	5.0	Striegel & Carpenter (1962)
Temik 10G	oral	not specified	rat	7.7	Weil (1973)
	dermal (4 h)	water	rat	400	Carpenter & Smyth (1965)
	dermal	none	rat	200	Carpenter & Smyth (1965)
	dermal	none	rat	850	Weil (1973)
	dermal	water (50%)	rabbit	32	West & Carpenter (1966)
	dermal (4 h)	dimethyl phthalate	rabbit	12.5	West & Carpenter (1966)
	dermal (4 h)	toluene (5%)	rabbit	3.5	West & Carpenter (1966)

[a] M = male; F = female.

acetylcholinesterase of a single feeding of aldicarb residues (about 83.4% sulfoxide and 16.6% sulfone). These residues were contained in a water-melon grown under experimental conditions, aldicarb having been applied to the soil at intervals beginning at the time of planting.

Water-melon with a residue concentration of 4.9 mg/kg was fed to three male and three female cynomolgus monkeys at a dosage that provided a residue intake of 0.005 mg/kg body weight. Additional groups of three male and three female monkeys received untreated water-melon (20 g/kg body weight). The test monkeys received supplemental untreated water-melon so that their total intake of the fruit was the same as that of the controls. Cholinesterase activity was measured 16, 9, and 3 days before and immediately before the test. Peak inhibition of plasma cholinesterase (31-46%) occurred 1 h after treatment. It was only slightly less at 2 h but was absent at 4 h after feeding. Observations continued at intervals for 24 h. No inhibition of erythrocyte cholinesterase and no clinical effects occurred (Trutter, 1989a).

A similar study with identical numbers of cynomolgus monkeys was conducted using treated bananas. The total residue level (0.25-0.29 mg/kg) in six bananas was less than that in the water-melon, and the average distribution of metabolites was different (91.8% sulfoxide and 8.2% sulfone). The dosage of aldicarb metabolites for the test monkeys was 0.005 mg/kg body weight and the banana intake for both test and control animals was 20 g/kg body weight. Inhibition of cholinesterase was similar in male and female test monkeys, averaging 23% one hour after dosing, increasing to 33% by the second hour, and decreasing to 24% by the fourth hour. No inhibition of erythrocyte cholinesterase and no clinical effects occurred (Trutter, 1989b).

7.2 Short-term exposure

Short-term studies have been conducted in several species with aldicarb and its principal metabolites (the sulfoxide and sulfone) both alone and in combination.

In studies by Weil & Carpenter (1968b,c), male and female rats were fed daily doses of aldicarb sulfoxide (0, 0.125, 0.25, 0.5, and 1.0 mg/kg body weight) or aldicarb sulfone (0, 0.2, 0.6, 1.8, 5.4, and 16.2 mg/kg body weight) in the diet for 3 and 6 months. Acetylcholinesterase activities were depressed at the three highest levels of each compound, and this was accompanied by some growth retardation. No mortality or pathological effects (gross or microscopic) were observed. In an earlier study, Weil & Carpenter (1963) fed male and female rats daily with 0, 0.02, 0.10, or 0.50 mg aldicarb/kg for 93 days. Plasma cholinesterase activity was depressed in both males and females but erythrocyte cholinesterase activity was depressed only in males. Male and female rats fed doses of either aldicarb sulfoxide or the sulfone (0.4, 1.0, 2.5, or 5.0 mg/kg body weight per day) for 7 days tolerated the lowest dose level of the sulfoxide with no effects on body or organ weight (Nycum & Carpenter, 1970). There was no evidence of plasma, erythrocyte or brain cholinesterase inhibition at that dose level. However, these parameters were significantly affected at all higher dose levels. Aldicarb sulfone caused a significant decrease in brain, plasma, and erythrocyte cholinesterase activity at the highest dose level in rats of both sexes. Reduction in brain cholinesterase activity also occurred at the two intermediate dose levels for the sulfone in female rats only.

In a 13-week feeding study (NCI, 1979), there was 100% mortality in rats exposed to 100 or 320 mg aldicarb/kg and body weight loss at 80 mg/kg in male rats.

DePass et al. (1985) exposed 8-week-old male and female Wistar rats (10 of each sex per group) to a 1:1 mixture of aldicarb sulfoxide and aldicarb sulfone in their drinking-water for 29 days. Their study was based on a report by Wilkinson et al. (1983) that residues of aldicarb in drinking-water consist essentially of a 1:1 mixture of the sulfoxide and sulfone. The drinking-water levels were 0, 0.075, 0.30, 1.20, 4.80, and 19.20 mg/litre (0–1.67 mg/kg body weight per day for males and 0–1.94 mg/kg body weight per day for females). The authors concluded that 4.8 mg/litre (470 µg/kg body weight per day) was the no-observed-effect level (NOEL), based on erythrocyte acetylcholinesterase and plasma cholinesterase inhibition observed at the highest dose level.

Short-term dermal studies were conducted in which Temik 10G (with 10% ai) was applied with wetted gauze to the abraded skin of male albino rabbits for 6 h/day for 15 days (Carpenter & Smyth, 1966). Dose levels of 0.05, 0.10, and 0.20 g/kg body weight were applied daily, and weight gain, food consumption, organ weights, cholinesterase activity, and the histopathology of several tissues were examined. Only plasma cholinesterase activity levels and weight gain at dose levels of 0.1 and 0.2 g/kg per day were significantly altered.

In a 2-year study on beagle dogs, aldicarb was administered in the diet at dose levels of 0, 0.025, 0.05, and 0.10 mg/kg body weight per day (Weil & Carpenter, 1966). The same parameters as those monitored in the rat study conducted by these authors were investigated in this study, but none were significantly different from controls. The authors concluded that the NOEL for rats and dogs was at least 0.10 mg/kg body weight per day, since this was the highest level tested.

In a study by Hamada (1988), male and female beagle dogs were fed for one year a diet containing 0, 1, 2, 5 or 10 mg technical aldicarb per kg to provide approximately 0, 0.025, 0.05, 0.13, or 0.25 mg/kg body weight per day. No dogs died during the study, and there were no effects on body weight, food and water consumption, organ weights, or on haematological, ophthalmological, histopathological, and gross pathological parameters. However, statistically significant increases, compared to controls, in the combined incidence of soft stools, mucoid stools, and diarrhoea were found in all groups treated with 0.05 mg/kg per day or more, as well as in females treated with 0.025 mg/kg per day. No statistically significant decrease in erythrocyte or brain cholinesterase was found in groups treated with 0.025 or 0.05 mg/kg body weight per day. However, plasma cholinesterase was inhibited in male dogs treated with 0.05 mg/kg body weight per day or more throughout the observation period of this study (weeks 5-52). In addition, plasma cholinesterase was inhibited at the conclusion of the study (week 52) in male dogs treated with 0.025 mg/kg body weight per day. The author noted that plasma cholinesterase activity in the male dogs treated with 0.025 mg/kg body weight per day was subsequently determined to be within historical control values, and that the statistically significant increase in soft stools and related effects in females treated with 0.025 mg/kg body weight per day could be attributable to an unusually high incidence of mucoid stools in one dog during the last half of the experiment. The author concluded that the NOEL in this study was 1 mg/kg (0.025 mg/kg body weight per day).

In a short-term study, Dorough et al. (1970) dosed lactating Holstein cows with Temik (10% ai) at 0.042 mg ai/kg body weight per day in their diet for 10 days and, in a second experiment, with a mixture of aldicarb and aldicarb sulfone (Temik equivalents of 0.006, 0.027, and 0.052 mg/kg body weight per day) for a period of 14 days. Although no alteration in blood cholinesterase activity levels or other clinical effects were noted, aldicarb sulfoxide and sulfone were detected in tissues. Milk production, feed consumption, and amount of excreta were unaltered.

7.3 Skin and eye irritation; sensitization

Pozzani & Carpenter (1968) observed that aldicarb (0.7 mg/kg body weight) in saline injected intradermally into male guinea-pigs had no sensitizing properties.

In male albino rabbits, application of aldicarb as a solution in propylene glycol on covered clipped skin did not produce any irritation. Instillation of 0.1 ml of a 25% suspension of aldicarb in propylene glycol or 1 mg of dry compound did not cause corneal irritation (Striegel & Carpenter, 1962).

The administration of 25 mg of aldicarb (Temik 5G) into the conjunctival sac of rabbits resulted in conjunctival irritation, which lasted for 24 h, in all the six test albino rabbits (Myers et al., 1983).

In a study by Myers et al. (1982), the application of 500 mg Temik 5G, moistened in saline solution, did not produce primary skin irritation in rabbits. Similarly percutaneous administration to abraded skin did not cause focal skin irritation.

Separate tests using aldicarb (75% wettable powder) and technical aldicarb in saline resulted in no sensitization response in male albino guinea-pigs following intradermal injections (Pozzani & Carpenter, 1968).

7.4 Long-term exposure

In a study by Weil & Carpenter (1972), male and female rats were fed aldicarb (0.3 mg/kg body weight per day), aldicarb sulfoxide (0.3 or 0.6 mg/kg body weight per day), aldicarb sulfone (0.6 or 2.4 mg/kg body weight/day), or a 1:1 mixture of the sulfoxide plus sulfone (0.6 or 1.2 mg/kg body weight per day) for 2 years. No effects were observed at the low dose level with any of the treatments. At the high dose level (except in the case of the sulfone), there was increased mortality within the first 30 days and a reduction in plasma cholinesterase activity, as well as decreased weight gain in the males. The NOEL values determined for aldicarb, aldicarb sulfoxide, aldicarb sulfone, and a 1:1 aldicarb sulfoxide/aldicarb sulfone mixture were 0.3, 0.3, 2.4, and 0.6 mg/kg body weight per day, respectively.

When male and female rats were fed diets containing aldicarb (0.005, 0.025, 0.05, or 0.1 mg/kg body weight per day) for 2 years, there were no effects on food consumption, mortality, lifespan, incidence of infection, liver and kidney weight, haematocrit, incidence of neoplasms and pathological lesions, or on plasma, brain, and erythrocyte cholinesterase levels (Weil & Carpenter, 1965).

7.5 Reproduction, embryotoxicity, and teratogenicity

Proctor et al. (1976) studied the effects of several methyl carbamate and organophosphate insecticides on teratogenicity and chicken embryo nicotinamide adenine dinucleotide (NAD) levels. Fertile White Leghorn eggs (45-55 g) were used for the test. After the eggs were incubated at 37 °C and 73% relative humidity for 4 or 5 days, 1 mg of aldicarb in a 30-μl methoxytriglycol solution was injected into the yolk and the injection hole on the shell was then sealed with paraffin wax. On day 12 after injection, some of the embryos were removed and the NAD levels were examined. On day 19 after injection, the remaining embryos (at least 10) were examined. NAD levels were similar to those of controls. There were no teratogenic effects (straight legs, abnormal feathers, or wry neck) in any of the embryos exposed to aldicarb.

In a study by Weil & Carpenter (1964), pregnant rats were fed with doses of 0, 0.04, 0.20, and 1.0 mg aldicarb per kg body weight per day. One group was fed throughout the pregnancy and until the pups were weaned, a second group was fed from the day of appearance of the vaginal plug until the 7th day of gestation, and a third group received aldicarb between days 5 and 15 of gestation. Although the highest dose administered was near the reported LD_{50} for rats, no significant effects on fertility, viability of offspring, lactation or other parameters were observed.

In a teratology study, Harlan-Wistar rats were fed aldicarb sulfone in their diets at dosages of 0.6, 2.4 or 9.6 mg/kg body weight per day, administered either during the first 20 days of gestation, during day 6 to day 15 of gestation, or during day 7 to day 9 of gestation. No treatment-related teratogenicity occurred as a result of any of the treatment regimes at any of the levels of exposure to the sulfone (Woodside et al., 1977).

Groups of 16 pregnant Dutch Belted rabbits were given doses of 0, 0.1, 0.25 or 0.50 mg aldicarb/kg body weight per day by gavage on days 7-27 of gestation (IRDC, 1983). Fetuses were then removed by Caesarean section. One spontaneous abortion was reported in each group given 0.25 or 0.50 mg/kg body weight per day. Although the number of viable fetuses and total implantation values were lower in all treatment groups than those in controls, they fell within historical control ranges and no significant differences were recorded.

Developmental toxicity of aldicarb has been evaluated by Tyl & Neeper-Bradley (1988). Four groups of pregnant CD Sprague-Dawley rats, 25 in each group, were administered aldicarb (0.125, 0.25 or 0.5 mg/kg body weight per day) in water solution by gavage from gestation days 6 to 15. There were three treatment-related maternal deaths in the high-dose group on day 7 of gestation (second day of administration). Maternal toxicity at that dose level was indicated by reduced body weight and food consumption and cholinergic signs. Body weight and food consumption were also reduced in the rats given 0.25 mg/kg body weight per day. The NOEL for maternal toxicity was 0.125 mg/kg body weight per day. Litter weight was significantly reduced at 0.5 mg/kg body weight per day. Fetotoxicity was indicated by body weight reduction, increased skeletal variation, retarded ossification, and ecchymosis on the trunk. No embryotoxicity was observed. An increased incidence of dilation of the cerebral lateral ventricle was observed at the highest dose level. However, due to the very high baseline control value for such changes found in pooled historical review, this increase was not considered to be significant.

In a 3-generation reproductive study on rats conducted by Weil & Carpenter (1964), aldicarb was incorporated into the diet of the parent generation at levels of 0.05 or 0.10 mg/kg body weight per day for 84 days before mating. Similar doses were fed to the subsequent F_2 and F_3 generations. No effects were noted.

In a further 3-generation reproductive toxicity study, Weil & Carpenter (1974a) fed Harlan-Wistar rats aldicarb in their diet at dosages of 0.2, 0.3 or 0.7 mg/kg body weight per day. No consistent treatment-related effects were observed in any of the parameters investigated.

A 3-generation reproductive toxicity study was performed on Harlan-Wistar rats that were fed aldicarb sulfone in their diets at levels adjusted to give dosages of 0.6, 2.4, and 9.6 mg/kg body weight per day (Woodside et al., 1977). Apart from occasional reductions in maternal body weight gain at the medium and high dosage levels, there were no treatment-related adverse effects on any of the parameters investigated.

Cambon et al. (1979) tested three carbamate insecticides (aldicarb, carbaferran, and primicarb) on acetylcholinesterase activity in tissues from pregnant Sprague-Dawley rats and fetuses. Aldicarb was administered by gastric intubation (0.001, 0.01 or 0.1 mg/kg body weight) to the pregnant animals (eight per group) on day 18 of gestation, and acetylcholinesterase activity was measured in maternal and fetal whole blood. Signs of poisoning occurred in animals about 5 min after the administration of the medium and high doses. There was significant inhibition of acetylcholinesterase in most maternal and fetal tissues, and its activity in maternal and fetal blood and liver was still lower than the control activity 24 h after treatment at the medium and high dose levels.

7.6 Mutagenicity and related end-points

Ercegovich & Rashid (1973) evaluated the mutagenicity of aldicarb in an Ames-type test using five strains of *Salmonella typhimurium* (identity of strains not stated). Aldicarb was found to be weakly mutagenic in the absence of a metabolic activation system.

Based on the results of four different laboratories that tested aldicarb for mutagenicity in *S. typhimurium* (TA98, TA100, TA1535, TA1537, and TA1538) and *E. coli* (WP2 *uvrA*), both with and without metabolic activation, Dunkel et al. (1985) reported that aldicarb did not produce a mutagenic response in any of the bacterial strains tested.

Rashid & Mumma (1986), reported that "technical grade aldicarb" (500 µg/plate) induced DNA damage in *S. typhimurium* (TA1538). It did not, however, have any lethal effect on the DNA-repair proficient strain of *S. typhimurium* (TA1978). No DNA-damage was caused in *E. coli* strains K-12 and WP2.

An *in vitro* gene mutation assay in L5178Y mouse lymphoma cells gave inconclusive results for aldicarb in the absence of metabolic activation, but aldicarb caused mutations in the presence of S9 mix from Aroclor 1254-induced F-344 rat liver (Myhr & Caspary, 1988). In an identical experiment performed at a different laboratory (Mitchell et al., 1988), aldicarb was shown to be mutagenic in both the presence and absence of induced S9 mix.

When aldicarb was tested *in vitro* in the CHO/HGPRT mammalian cell forward gene mutation assay, there was no evidence of mutagenicity either in the presence or absence of S9 mix from Aroclor 1254-induced male Sprague-Dawley rat livers (Stankowski et al., 1985).

Blevins et al. (1977) found no evidence of DNA damage in human skin fibroblasts exposed *in vitro* to aldicarb.

No evidence that aldicarb caused any unscheduled DNA synthesis in primary cultures of hepatocytes from male F-344 rats was detected by Godek et al. (1984).

Aldicarb caused increases in the numbers of chromatid and chromosome breaks in human peripheral lymphocytes exposed *in vitro* (Cid & Matos, 1987). This effect was greater in the presence of S9 mix from phenobarbital-induced livers of male Sprague-Dawley rats than in its absence.

When Cid & Matos (1984) studied the effects of aldicarb on human lymphocytes *in vitro*, they found that it caused a significant increase in sister chromatid exchanges (SCE). Slightly higher SCE values were found in the presence of S9 liver homogenate fractions than in its absence.

The *in vivo* clastogenicity of aldicarb in bone marrow has been investigated in rats and mice via the intraperitoneal route. Sharaf et al. (1982) treated male albino rats (strain not stated) with injections of aldicarb (0.00121, 0.00666 or 0.0121 mg/kg body weight) dissolved in a 1:1 water/acetone vehicle. One group of animals served as a control, a second group received one injection per day for 5 days, and a third group received one injection only. Increases in structural and numerical aberrations were observed in bone marrow cells in all groups of treated animals. Structural chromosomal aberrations consisted of chromatid breaks or deletions, chromatid gaps, centromeric attenuation, and (in the case of repeated exposure only) centric fusions. Numerical aberrations were mainly due to endomitosis, although there was also some evidence of increased polyploidy. In mice, however, there was no evidence of any effect on chromosomal aberration frequencies in bone marrow cells following a single intraperitoneal injection of aldicarb (93.5% pure; 0.010 or 0.001 mg/kg body weight). In addition, no effects were seen when five daily doses of 0.010 mg/kg body weight were given (Cimmino et al., 1984).

Dominant lethal studies have been performed using Harlan-Wistar rats (from the F_2 generation of multigeneration studies) that had been treated with aldicarb (Weil & Carpenter, 1974a) or aldicarb sulfone (Woodside et al., 1977) given in the diet at dosages of 0.2, 0.3, and 0.7 mg/kg (aldicarb) and 0.6, 2.4, and 9.6 mg/kg (aldicarb sulfone). The treated males were then mated with untreated virgin females. The results of the studies gave no indication of an increased incidence of dominant lethal mutations in rats treated orally with aldicarb or aldicarb sulfone.

Although some of the mutagenicity tests performed on aldicarb gave positive results, the results of the various *in vitro* and *in vivo* tests, when considered together, indicate that aldicarb is not an *in vivo* mutagen.

The mutagenic potential of N-nitroso aldicarb has also been investigated. A bacterial spot test conducted with *Salmonella typhimurium* his$^-$ G46 gave a weakly positive result (Seiler, 1977). Blevins et al. (1977) investigated the interaction of N-nitroso aldicarb with DNA in *in vitro* human skin fibroblasts and found numerous single-strand breaks in the DNA of all the nitroso-derivative-treated cells but not in the DNA from cells treated with aldicarb itself. Cid et al. (1988) found that N-nitroso-aldicarb caused an increase in the number of sister chromatid exchanges in human lymphocytes *in vitro*.

7.7 Carcinogenicity

Weil (1968) reported a skin-painting study of male mice in which a 0.125% solution of aldicarb was applied to the hair-free skin on the backs of animals twice a week for up to 28 months. There were no substantial differences with respect to the incidence of tumours. Two growths, a haemangioma and a thymoma, were noted in the animals administered aldicarb. These internal growths were not accompanied by cutaneous papillomas or carcinomas and were considered to be spontaneous growths unrelated to any incidence of malignancy (Wilkinson et al., 1983).

In a study by Weil & Carpenter (1974b), aldicarb was dissolved in acetone prior to mixing with the diet, and dietary levels of 0.1, 0.3 or 0.7 mg/kg body weight were administered to groups of 50 male CD-1 mice for 18 months. Two control groups of 50 mice were used in addition to a group of untreated mice from which one animal was killed for comparison purposes each time a mouse in the aldicarb-treated groups died during the experimental period. There was no treatment-related effect on mortality. Furthermore, there were no treatment-related effects on the incidence of any tumour type at any site or on the total incidence of tumours.

In a study by Woodside et al. (1977), groups of CD-1 mice (50 of each sex per group) were administered aldicarb sulfone (0, 0.15, 0.6, 2.4 or 9.6 mg/kg body weight) in the food for 18 months. Observations included mortality, food consumption, and body weight determinations, and gross and microscopic examinations were performed on all mice. Body weight changes were sporadic and exhibited no trends. Histological changes were not statistically different from those in controls at any dose level for either sex.

In a 2-year feeding study on rats, Weil & Carpenter (1965, 1972) reported no significant tumour increases in rats fed aldicarb (0.005, 0.025, 0.05, 0.10, or 0.30 mg/kg body weight per day) or its sulfoxide and sulfone. In an NCI (1979) bioassay, male and female F-344 rats and $B6C3F_1$ mice were given technical aldicarb (2 or 6 mg/kg body weight) in their diet for 103 weeks. No treatment-related tumours were observed in either species.

Quarles et al. (1979) performed a series of experiments to examine the transforming and tumorigenic activity of aldicarb and its nitroso derivative. Pregnant hamsters were given intraperitoneal injections of aldicarb (0.1 or 0.5 mg/kg) or nitroso-aldicarb (2 mg/kg) on day 10 of gestation. Fetal cell cultures were prepared and plated on agar on day 13 of gestation. To test for tumorigenicity, 1×10^6 cells were injected subcutaneously into adult nude mice. Aldicarb was found to be inactive and did not induce either morphological transformations or cells that grew in agar, whereas nitroso-aldicarb induced morphological transformations that were tumorigenic in nude mice.

Weekly administration by oral gavage of N-nitroso-aldicarb (nine doses of 10 mg/kg body weight or two doses of 20 mg/kg body weight) to groups of 12 female Sprague-Dawley rats resulted in the development, by the end of their natural lives, of forestomach carcinomas in two of the rats from each treated group, compared with none in control animals (Lijinsky & Schmahl, 1978). The nitroso derivative of aldicarb may be formed in the laboratory when aldicarb is in the presence of nitrite under the pH and temperature conditions of the human stomach (Elespuru & Lijinsky, 1973; Lijinsky & Schmahl, 1978).

7.8 Other special studies

Farage-Elawar (1988) studied the functional consequences of dosing six-day-old chicks orally with 0.2 mg aldicarb/kg body weight per day for seven days. Both acetylcholinesterase and neuropathy target esterase levels were determined during treatment and on days 1, 3, 6, 10, 20, 30, and 40 after treatment. Measurements of motor function consisted of analysis of the gait at the same times. Six days after the last treatment there was a significant weight reduction with no recovery to the control weight. There were significant alterations in three parameters of gait starting on post-treatment day 1 and lasting until day 40. Aldicarb reduced the acetylcholinesterase levels significantly only 24 h after the first day of treatment, with recovery to control levels thereafter. There were no significant alterations in neuropathy target esterase levels at any time. The authors concluded that motor function changes in the young chick can be seen in the absence of alterations in acetylcholinesterase levels.

Olsen et al. (1987) conducted studies using low concentrations of aldicarb (0, 1, 10, 100 or 1000 µg per litre) in the drinking-water of inbred Swiss Webster mice for 34 days and measured the splenic plaque-forming cells (PFC) response to sheep red blood cells. The mean PFC count in the 1-µg/litre group was significantly less than in the control group after 34 days. The authors stated that aldicarb exhibited immunomodulatory capability.

Thomas et al. (1987) conducted experiments similar to Olson et al. (1987), but used both Swiss Webster and $B6C3F_1$ mice. The mean PFC counts at 0.1 µg/litre were lower than the controls; at 1.0 µg/litre they exceeded the controls; and at 10 µg/litre they were lower than the controls. With $B6C3F_1$ mice PFC counts exceeded control values at both 100 and 1000 µg/litre, whereas in the case of Swiss Webster mice they were similar to control values at 100 µg/litre but lower at 1000 µg/litre. The authors concluded that aldicarb at environmentally relevant exposure concentrations is not immunotoxic in rodents.

Shirazi et al. (1990) studied the immunomodulation response of mice to low levels of aldicarb in drinking-water (0.01 to 1000 µg/litre). Compared to the mean PFC values of the control group, the mean values of treated groups indicated a stimulatory effect for 30- and 60-day tests and an inhibitory effect for 90- and 180-days tests. However, when the data were reanalysed using the distribution of the relative PFC counts, a consistently inhibitory response was observed. The authors concluded that the dose-response relationships indicated a polyphasic and inhibitory response.

Selvan et al. (1989) observed that aldicarb selectively affected macrophage-mediated cytotoxicity of tumor target cells without affecting the cytotoxicity mediated by natural killer cells. However, no dose-response relationship was found.

Dean et al. (1990) investigated the effect of aldicarb on syngenic mixed lymphocyte reaction (SMLR). In this reaction $CD4^+$ T-helper cells (autoreactive T cells) respond to syngenic Ia molecules expressed on C3H mouse macrophages. The authors reported that intraperitoneal treatment (0.1 ml per mouse of a solution containing 0.1 to 1000 µg aldicarb per litre) suppressed the SMLR by selectively decreasing the stimulatory activity of macrophages without affecting directly the responsiveness of autoreactive T cells.

A significant suppression of macrophage-mediated cytotoxicity of tumor cells was observed in C3H mice that received seven daily doses of 0.1 to 10 µg aldicarb per kg. The authors concluded that aldicarb may selectively affect the macrophage function but not directly affect other components of the immune response.

Thomas & Ratajczak (1988) reported that when aldicarb was administered in the drinking-water (0.1, 1.0, 10, 100 or 1000 µg/litre) *ad libitum* for 34 consecutive days to both Swiss Webster and $B6C3F_1$ hybrid female mice, there were no effects in either strain on body weight, organ weight, circulatory white blood cells or microscopic pathology of the thymus, spleen, liver, kidneys or lymph nodes. *In vivo* host resistance to infectious viral challenge was unaffected by aldicarb treatment. Aldicarb was found to have no effect in either strain on the number of antibody-forming cells in the spleen or on the amount of circulating antibody in the blood. The capacity of B and T lymphocytes to respond to nonspecific mitogens was unaltered, as was the ability of T lymphocytes to recognize genetically different cell types in a mixed lymphocyte culture (MLC). It was concluded that aldicarb in drinking-water had no effect on any measured immunological function.

Thomas et al. (1990) exposed adult female $B6C3F_1$ mice to drinking-water containing 1.0, 10 or 100 µg aldicarb per litre or to distilled drinking-water alone for 34 consecutive days. The impact of aldicarb exposure on the ability of splenic natural killer cells and specifically sensitized cytotoxic T lymphocytes to lyse YAC-1 lymphoma target cells and P 815 tumor cells was evaluated. The percentages and absolute numbers of total T cells, T-suppressor, T-helper, and B cells was also measured. The authors concluded that the absence of statistically significant effects on any of these parameters indicated that aldicarb treatment did not adversely affect the immune system of mice.

7.9 Factors modifying toxicity; toxicity of metabolites

Of the metabolites that have been identified, only the sulfoxide and sulfone have a mechanism of toxicity similar to aldicarb (as a cholinesterase inhibitor in a carbamylation reaction). The sulfoxide appears to be equally toxic and the sulfone considerably less toxic than aldicarb in acute and long-term tests (Weil, 1968; Weil & Carpenter, 1972).

7.10 Mechanisms of toxicity - mode of action

Aldicarb and acetylcholine exhibit very close structural similarity.

$$CH_3S-\underset{\underset{CH_3}{|}}{\overset{\overset{CH_3}{|}}{C}}-CH=N-O\overset{O}{\overset{\|}{C}}NHCH_3 \qquad CH_3-\underset{\underset{CH_3}{|}}{\overset{\overset{CH_3}{|}}{N}}-CH_2CH_2O\overset{O}{\overset{\|}{C}}CH_3$$

Aldicarb   Acetylcholine

The mechanism of toxic action of aldicarb and its metabolites (sulfoxide and sulfone) involves their reaction with cholinesterase enzymes. In particular, the carbamylation of acetylcholinesterase interferes with hydrolysis of acetylcholine at synaptic and myoneural junctions. This adversely affects neural transmission (Carpenter & Smyth, 1965; Weil & Carpenter, 1968a,b,c, 1970; Dorough, 1970). Various cholinesterase enzymes have been identified in the plasma, red blood cells, liver, and brain (Kuhr & Dorough, 1976; Cambon et al., 1980). The function of plasma cholinesterase is not fully understood, but it is considered to play no role in cholinergic transmission. Acetylcholinesterase in erythrocytes reflects the acetylcholinesterase activity in the nerve synapses. Since acetylcholinesterase in erythrocytes and in nerve synapses are considered to be biochemically identical, erythrocyte cholinesterase activity may be taken as an indicator of the biochemical effect of anti-cholinesterase pesticides (WHO, 1990a).

Carbamates, like organophosphates, inhibit esterases (serine-esterases and/or beta-esterases) (WHO, 1986). Although the inhibition of serine-esterases other than acetylcholinesterase is not significant for the toxicity of the compound, it may have significance for the potentiation of toxicity of other compounds after long-term low level exposure (Sakai & Matsumara, 1968, 1971; Aldridge & Magos 1978). The site of carbamylation of the enzyme is the hydroxyl moiety of the serine amino acid. The rate of reactivation of the carbamylated enzyme to acetylcholinesterase is relatively rapid compared to that of the enzyme phosphorylated by an organophosphorus pesticide. Thus the inhibition of acetylcholinesterase by carbamate pesticides is rapid and reversible. The chemistry of carbamate pesticides is such that no aging reaction is possible, as occurs with the phosphorylated enzyme. In order to permit an evaluation of cholinesterase inhibition by carbamates *in vivo*, special care is required. Carbamate cholinesterase inhibition studies should utilize minimal dilution during the preparation of the assay, minimal incubation times, and minimal time between blood sampling and assay (WHO, 1990a).

8. EFFECTS ON HUMANS

8.1 General population exposure

The symptoms that have been reported for accidental or occupational poisoning and controlled human exposure to aldicarb are cholinergic and subside spontaneously, usually within 6 h, unless death intervenes. Clinical symptoms and signs include dizziness, salivation, excessive sweating, nausea, epigastric cramps, vomiting, diarrhoea, bronchial secretion, blurred vision, non-reactive contracted pupils, dyspnoea, and muscular fasciculations. The intensity of these symptoms varies with the extent of exposure.

8.1.1 Acute toxicity; poisoning incidents

The first reported case of accidental poisoning occurred in 1966 when aldicarb was being used as an experimental pesticide (Hayes, 1982). The wife of an experimental scientist used a small amount of a 10% granular formulation to treat the soil around a rose bush. Twenty-four days later she ate a sprig of mint from a plant growing nearby, which consisted of the terminal 4-6 leaves and the stem. Thirty minutes later she vomited and had diarrhoea and involuntary urination. On admission to the hospital, she was found to have pinpoint pupils, muscle fasciculations, and difficulty in breathing. Maximal signs were observed 2 h after onset. She was given 1 mg of atropine with no observable effect. About 15 min later she was given 2 mg atropine and had transient opening of the pupils. A further 2 mg atropine was followed by sustained opening of the pupils and gradual improvement in the patient's condition. Three-and-a-half hours after onset, she was resting comfortably and had no further signs or symptoms. It was estimated that she had eaten between 0.5 and 1.0 g of mint. Feeding 3.0 g of this mint to a rabbit resulted in its death within 2 h; 2.4 g caused severe symptoms in a second rabbit.

Two minor incidents of aldicarb poisoning with moderately severe symptoms occurred after hydroponically grown cucumbers were eaten (CDC, 1979; Goes et al., 1980; Hayes,

1982). Although carbamates had been used in both cases, there were no data on the aldicarb content of the cucumbers in the first case. Levels of 6.6-10.7 mg aldicarb/kg were found in the second case (the hydroponic nutrient solution contained 1.8 mg aldicarb/litre). The symptoms lasted only 4.5-6.0 h, and recovery from cholinergic symptoms occurred without specific treatment (Aaronson et al., 1979).

Aldicarb food poisoning from contaminated melons was reported in California, USA, in 1985. Of the 1358 cases reported, 692 were classified as probable. The melons were tested for aldicarb sulfoxide, and 10 (4%) of the 250 tests were positive. The most severe signs and symptoms included loss of consciousness and cardiac arrhythmia. Six deaths and two stillbirths were reported but no analyses for aldicarb sulfoxide were reported (Jackson et al., 1986; Ting & Kho, 1986).

Goldman et al. (1990a) analysed the same epidemic in California in 1985. According to their result, 1376 cases of illness within California were reported to the California Department of Health Services of which 77% were classified as being probably or possible carbamate-related illnesses. Seventeen individuals required hospitalization.

An outbreak of illness caused by aldicarb-contaminated water-melons was reported in Oregon, USA, in 1985. About 264 cases of poisoning were reported and 61 definite cases were confirmed. The levels of residue in the water-melons ranged from 0.01 mg/kg (limit of detection) to 6.3 mg/kg. (Green et al., 1987).

Goldman et al. (1990b) reviewed three outbreaks of poisoning due to aldicarb-contaminated water-melons or cucumbers in California between 1985 and 1988, and one outbreak due to contaminated cucumbers in England. Estimated dosages of aldicarb sulfoxide that caused the illnesses ranged between 0.0011 and 0.06 mg/kg body weight and most were well below the 0.025 mg/kg for subclinical whole blood cholinesterase depression.

Ramasamy (1976) reported an incident in which a 7-month-old female baby ate some aldicarb powder. Recovery was complete after she was given a total dose of 105.6 mg atropine.

8.1.2 Human studies

An experimental study was carried out on 12 men already involved in the study of aldicarb and, therefore, familiar with its effects. Four volunteers in each of three groups took aldicarb (99.2% purity; dissolved in drinking-water) at concentrations of 0.025, 0.05, or 0.10 mg/kg body weight. Blood was collected for cholinesterase measurement at 18 h and 1 h before ingestion of aldicarb and at 1, 2, 4, and 6 h after ingestion. The samples of whole blood were analysed by the radiometric method for whole blood, which has the advantage of involving minimal dilution of the blood and a maximum of only 3 min from the time the sample is taken until the chemical reaction is complete (the period of storage of the samples until the radioactivity in them is measured has no effect on the result). The compound hydrolysed is acetylcholine and not, as in many methods, a substitute. Urine samples were collected at 1, 2, 4, and 6 h after ingestion. Analysis was by gas chromatography after all metabolites had been oxidized to aldicarb sulfone. The highest dosage chosen was that already found to be a no-observed-effect level in a 2-year rat feeding study. This was done even though it was recognized that some symptoms might occur if ingestion occupied less than 1 min rather than 24 h as in the rat. Signs and symptoms did, in fact, occur at the highest dosage and included nausea and vomiting, pinpoint non-reactive pupils, malaise, weakness, epigastric pain, air hunger and yawning, sweating of the hands, forearms and forehead, salivation, and slurred speech. The authors stated that none of the signs and symptoms were severe and they required no treatment. Cholinesterase activity was depressed in proportion to the dosage. Based on the individual 18-h pre-dosing samples, the average level 1 h after ingestion was reduced to 53.3, 38.8, and 34.6% of normal at 0.025, 0.05, and 0.1 mg/kg, respectively. At the highest dosage, the activity was further decreased (28.1% of normal) in the 2-h sample, but it was elevated at the two lower dosages. At 4 h it was elevated in all groups but by 6 h it had almost returned to normal. Urinary excretion of metabolites was proportional to dosage; the total recovery varied from 3.4 to 10.7% during the 8 h (Haines, 1971).

Effects on Humans

In a separate test of volunteers, one man took a dosage of 0.26 mg/kg body weight in the form of Temik 10G granules. He became ill and took atropine. The carbamate concentration was greatest in a urine sample collected 4.5 h after ingestion, but total recovery of aldicarb was only 8.1% in 24 h (Cope & Romine, 1973).

8.1.3 Epidemiological studies

After aldicarb had been detected in well-water samples in Suffolk County, New York, Varma et al. (1983) conducted a preliminary mail survey of families who had consumed water from these wells in 1981. The 1500 subjects had consumed water that contained from 8 to over 64 µg aldicarb/litre. They were asked to report any symptoms of 20 general health problems and the outcome of all pregnancies. A list of 25 randomly arranged neurological symptoms was also included. The response rate (20%) was poor. No conclusive evidence of the association of health problems with aldicarb exposure was obtained from this study (for which there were no controls), although there appeared to be an association between some neurological symptoms/syndromes and the concentration of aldicarb in the well water. The rate of spontaneous abortions was also high among women who consumed water from wells that contained the highest aldicarb concentrations (66 µg/litre or more).

In a cross-sectional study of exposed and unexposed residents of Portage County, Wisconsin, Fiore et al. (1986) reported the effects of chronic ingestion of ground water contaminated with levels of aldicarb (< 61 µg per litre) on the immune function of 50 women aged 18 to 70 with no known underlying reason for immunodysfunction. Of these exposed women, 23 consumed water from a source with detectable levels of aldicarb, while 27 unexposed women consumed water from a source with no detectable level of aldicarb. Exposed women showed an elevated stimulation assay response to Candida antigen, an increase in the number of T8 cells, and a decrease in the ratio of T4:T8 cells as compared with unexposed women. Although the results of this study are of interest, the T lymphocyte data fall within the normal range indicated by Martin et al. (1985). The Candida response data are also within normal limits that have been routinely observed at the University of Wisconsin Medical Center. The results of this study, because of the presence of other contaminants, present no evidence for a causal relationship between consumption of water contaminated with aldicarb and alteration of immunological parameters.

8.2 Occupational exposure

8.2.1 Acute toxicity; poisoning incidents

Peoples et al. (1978) reported on occupational exposure to aldicarb in California during the period 1974-1976. They reviewed 38 illnesses, 31 of which were systemic, that were directly related to occupational aldicarb (Temik) exposure. There were four cases of contact dermatitis and one case of eye irritation in which dust from Temik granules was blown directly into the eye causing chemical conjunctivitis.

Lee & Ransdell (1984) reported the death of a 20-year-old farm worker who was run over by a tractor after he had been handling Temik 15G. Tissue samples taken at autopsy revealed an estimated body burden of 18.2 mg aldicarb (0.275 mg/kg). This level is nearly 3 times higher than that known to produce cholinergic symptoms in humans, and the authors considered that pesticide intoxication contributed to the worker's death.

Sexton (1966) reported the incapacitation of a foreman working in an aldicarb mechanical bagging operation. Symptoms of cholinesterase depression lasted longer than 6 h, but he returned to work the next day. Griffith & Duncan (1985) surveyed Florida citrus fruit growers over a 12-month period for aldicarb-related poisonings. Only one case, that of a certified applicator who required hospitalization for cholinergic symptoms, was directly related to the aldicarb exposure.

Aldicarb is one of the most potent and acutely toxic pesticides in use. In most cases, excessive occupational exposure to aldicarb has been due either to its improper application or to the improper use of protective equipment. Its formulation as granules and its application to the subsoil as a systemic pesticide have been recommended

Effects on Humans

by the manufacturer to reduce the hazards (SR1, 1984).

8.2.2 *Effects of short- and long-term exposure; epidemiological studies*

No controlled occupational exposure or epidemiological studies have been reported.

9. EFFECTS ON OTHER ORGANISMS IN THE LABORATORY AND FIELD

9.1 Microorganisms

Some aspects of the effects of microorganisms on aldicarb have been discussed in section 4.3.1. In the study by Kuseske et al. (1974), application rates of 5 and 500 ppm of a commercial formulation of aldicarb (100 g/kg ai) caused a decrease in the population of microflora for the first 16 days and then stimulated the population growth, in proportion to the application rate, over the next 14 days. The microorganisms used in this study were *Actinomycetes*, *Nitrosomonas europaea*, and *Nitrobacter agilis*. When 5 ppm of the insecticide was applied, depletion of *Nitrosomonas* resulted in complete inhibition of the conversion of the ammonium ion to nitrite. The oxidative capability of five common soil fungi (Jones, 1976) is discussed in section 4.3.1. Spurr & Sousa (1966, 1967) found no inhibition of bacterial or fungal growth by aldicarb. Indeed, in the case of *Rhizoctonia solani* (a plant pathogen and soil saprophyte), the addition of aldicarb to the medium doubled its growth rate. The authors concluded that microorganisms probably used aldicarb as a carbon source.

9.2 Aquatic organisms

The acute toxicity of aldicarb to freshwater aquatic organisms varies greatly. The 96-h LC_{50} values for different species of fish range between 52 and 2420 µg per litre at different temperatures and water hardness (Table 10). Aquatic molluses are very insensitive to the effects of aldicarb (Singh & Agarwal, 1981). For the adult water flea, *Daphnia laevis*, the sulfoxide is more toxic than aldicarb by a factor of two and the sulfone less toxic by a factor of five to six (Foran et al., 1985). For the bluegill sunfish, *Lepomis macrochirus*, the toxicity of aldicarb and the sulfoxide is comparable, but the sulfone is less toxic (Clarkson, 1968b). For estuarine and marine organisms, acute lethality is less variable with 96-h LC_{50} values ranging between 13 and 170 µg/litre for all species tested (Table 10). Pant & Kumar (1981) studied

Table 10. Acute toxicity (LC_{50}) of aldicarb to freshwater, estuarine, and marine organisms[a]

Organism	Age/size	Stat/flow	M/N	Temperature (°C)	Hardness (mg/litre)	pH	Compound	Duration	Concentration (μg/litre)	Reference
Freshwater species										
Water flea (Daphnia laevis)	adult	stat	M	21	58	6.9	A	48 h	209 (175-265)	Foran et al. (1985)
			M	21	58	6.9	AX	48 h	103 (36-142)	Foran et al. (1985)
			M	21	58	6.9	AN	48 h	1124 (993-1320)	Foran et al. (1985)
	juvenile (1-3 days old)						A		70 (61-84)	Foran et al. (1985)
							AX		84 (73-95)	Foran et al. (1985)
							AN		910 (821-1099)	Foran et al. (1985)
Water flea (Daphnia magna)							A	48 h	410	US EPA (1988a)
Water snail (Lymnaea acuminata)	adult	stat					A	24 h	30 000	Singh & Agarwal (1981)
								96 h	11 500	Singh & Agarwal (1981)
								240 h	7500	Singh & Agarwal (1981)
Water snail (Pila globosa)	adult	stat					A	96 h	175 000	Singh & Agarwal (1981)
								240 h	78 000	Singh & Agarwal (1981)
Bluegill sunfish (Lepomis macrochirus)	1.3 g	stat		24	44	7.4	A	24 h	103 (66-161)	Mayer & Ellersieck (1986)
	1.3 g	stat		24	44	7.4	A	96 h	52 (34-79)	Mayer & Ellersieck (1986)
	3.9 g	stat		18	44	7.4	A	24 h	160 (130-214)	Mayer & Ellersieck (1986)
	3.9 g	stat		18	44	7.4	A	96 h	71 (54-93)	Mayer & Ellersieck (1986)
	5.0 g	stat					A	72 h	100	Clarkson (1968b)
	5.0 g	stat					AX	72 h	4000	Clarkson (1968b)
	5.0 g	stat					AN	72 h	64 000	Clarkson (1968b)
Rainbow trout (Salmo gairdneri)	0.5 g	stat		12	44	7.4	A	24 h	1000 (727-1376)	Mayer & Ellersieck (1986)
	0.5 g	stat		12	44	7.4	A	96 h	560 (394-796)	Mayer & Ellersieck (1986)
	2.7 g	stat		18	44	7.4	A	24 h	780 (592-1027)	Mayer & Ellersieck (1986)
	2.7 g	stat		18	44	7.4	A	96 h	660 (472-921)	Mayer & Ellersieck (1986)
Barbus conchonius	4.8 cm	stat		14-22	319	7.4	A	48 h	8990 (4265-18 586)	Pant & Kumar (1981)
	4.8 cm	stat		14-22	319	7.4	A	96 h	2420 (2280-2520)	Pant & Kumar (1981)
	4.8 cm	stat		14-22	61	7.2	A	48 h	3296 (1116-9727)	Pant & Kumar (1981)
	4.8 cm	stat		14-22	61	7.2	A	96 h	459 (445-521)	Pant & Kumar (1981)

Table 10 (contd).

Organism	Age/size	Stat/flow	M/N	Temperature (°C)	Salinity °/oo	pH	Compound	Duration	Concentration (µg/litre)	Reference
Estuarine & marine species										
Alga (*Skeletonema costatum*)		stat	N	20	30		A	96 h	> 50 000[b]	Mayer (1987)
Mysid shrimp (*Mysidopsis bahia*)	juvenile (1 day old)	stat	N	25	20		A	96 h	13 (10-15)	Mayer (1987)
	adult	flow	M	22	28		A	96 h	16 (13-20)	Mayer (1987)
Pink shrimp (*Penaeus duorarum*)	adult	flow	M	22	29		A	96 h	12 (7.5-18)	Mayer (1987)
White shrimp (*Penaeus stylirostris*)	juvenile	stat	N	25	20		A	96 h	72 (65-82)	Mayer (1987)
Eastern oyster (*Crassostrea virginica*)	embryo	stat	N	25	20		A	48 h	8800[c] (1400-56 000)	Mayer (1987)
Sheepshead minnow (*Cyprinodon variegatus*)	juvenile (28 days old)	stat	N	25	20		A	96 h	170 (100-320)	Mayer (1987)
	adult	flow	M	28	28		A	96 h	41 (55-72)	Mayer (1987)
Pinfish (*Lagodon rhomboides*)	adult	flow	M	22	30		A	96 h	80 (43-150)	Mayer (1987)
Spot (*Leiostomus xanthurus*)	adult	stat	N	25	20		A	96 h	200 (120-290)	Mayer (1987)
Snook (*Centropomus undecimalis*)	juvenile (0.23 g)	stat	N	26-30	35		A	48 h	100	Landau & Tucker (1984)

[a] M = measured concentration; N = nominal concentration; stat = static conditions; flow = flow-through conditions; A = aldicarb; AX = aldicarb sulfoxide; AN = aldicarb sulfone. [b] LC$_{50}$ for growth. [c] LC$_{50}$ for metamorphosis.

the acute toxicity of aldicarb to the Himalayan lake teleost *Barbus conchonius* in both hard and soft water. Temperatures varied from 14 to 22 °C during the experiment, and the tests were carried out under static conditions. Results indicated that the toxicity of aldicarb to *B. conchonius* was considerably greater in soft water (Table 10). Mortality data showed that concentrations of 1.5 mg/litre in soft water and 6.0 mg/litre in hard water resulted in 100% mortality within 96 h.

Landau & Tucker (1984) exposed eggs of the estuarine snook *(Centropomus undecimalis)* from 2 to 3 h after fertilization to various aldicarb concentrations. Larvae were more sensitive than eggs to aldicarb. Mortality over 14 to 25 h was 0, 17, 22, and 30% of embryos and 0, 83, 78, and 70% of larvae at 0.025, 0.1, 0.25, and 0.5 mg per litre, respectively.

Pickering & Gilliam (1982) exposed eggs and newly hatched larvae of the freshwater fathead minnow to aldicarb at 20, 38, 78, 156, and 340 µg/litre and monitored hatching and growth of juveniles over 30 days. None of the aldicarb concentrations affected embryo survival and only the two highest levels reduced larval-juvenile survival (by 58% and 80%, respectively) over 30 days. Growth of surviving young was reduced significantly only at the highest exposure concentration. Based on the acute maximum acceptable toxic concentration (MATC) of 78 to 156 µg per litre, the authors calculated a chronic MATC of 110 µg aldicarb/litre.

9.3 Terrestrial organisms

Haque & Ebing (1983) conducted a 14-day laboratory toxicity test of aldicarb using the earthworms *Lumbricus terrestris* and *Eisenia foetida* as test species. The pesticide was homogeneously incorporated into the test soil substrates. The authors noted a species-specific variation in toxicity, *L. terrestris* showing an LC_{50} of 530 (490-565) and *E. foetida* of 65 (58-75) mg/kg dry soil substrate.

The acute oral LD_{50} for birds has been found to vary between 0.8 and 5.3 mg/kg body weight, while the dietary toxicity ranged from approximately 250 to 800 mg/kg diet

(Table 11). West & Carpenter (1965) reported that the oral LD_{50} for White Leghorn cockerels was 9 mg/kg body weight (i.e. 10 times that of rats). Symptoms of aldicarb poisoning in chickens were excessive salivation, dyspnoea, stiffness, and twitching of leg, wing, and pectoral muscles (Schlinke, 1970). When 28-day-old Japanese quail (*Coturnix coturnix japonica*) were given analytical grade aldicarb in corn oil solution (in gelatin capsules) at a dose of 30 mg/kg body weight (i.e. 3 times the LD_{50}), all birds died within 3 h (Martin et al., 1981). Balcomb et al. (1984) measured the acute oral toxicity of aldicarb to two species of song bird (house sparrow and redwinged blackbird) (Table 11). When birds were dosed with varying numbers of aldicarb granules (Temik 15G), 40% of blackbirds given a single granule died, and 80% of those given 5 granules died. In a study on the redwinged blackbird, technical and granular (Temik 15G) aldicarb yielded similar LD_{50} values. However, the oral LD_{50} of granular aldicarb for sparrows was 3.8 mg/kg body weight whereas that for technical aldicarb was 0.8 mg/kg/body weight. Hill & Camardese (1981) reported that dietary LC_{50} values in young Japanese quail *(Coturnix coturnix japonica)* increased with the age of the bird, the increase being reasonably predictable between 7 and 21 days of age. Five-day dietary LC_{50} values were 247, 355, 542, and 786 mg/kg diet at ages 1, 7, 14, and 21 days, respectively.

In studies by Schlinke (1970) on the toxic effects of aldicarb and other nematocides in chickens, groups of five White Leghorn chickens, 6-7 weeks old, were given oral doses of 1.0, 2.5 or 5 mg aldicarb/kg per day. Individual doses were administered in gelatin capsules or by an aqueous oral drench for 10 days. Groups of six to eight chickens were used simultaneously as controls. Body weight gain and mortality were determined. In the low-dose group, a slight decrease in the percentage body weight gain (44% treated versus 49% controls) was observed, but no adverse effects were reported at this level. Body weight gain for the chickens given 2.5 mg/kg was 30% versus 40% in controls. In addition one chicken died after receiving a single dose of the compound and a second died after receiving three consecutive daily doses. In the high-dose groups (5 mg/kg per day), one chicken died after receiving a single dose (day 1 of administration), one after the

Table 11. Oral and dietary toxicity of aldicarb to birds

Species	Age	Exposure[a]	Parameter	Concentration (mg/kg)[b]	Reference
House sparrow (*Passer domesticus*)	adult	oral	LD_{50}	0.8	Balcomb et al. (1984)
Redwinged blackbird (*Agelaius phoenicus*)	adult	oral	LD_{50}	1.8	Balcomb et al. (1984)
Grackle (*Quiscalus quiscula*)		oral	LD_{50}	0.8	d
Starling (*Sturnus vulgaris*)		oral	LD_{50}	4.2	d
Pigeon (*Columba livia* var.)		oral	LD_{50}	3.2	d
California quail (*Lophortyx californica*)	10 months	oral	LD_{50}	M: 2.6 (2-3.4) F: 4.7 (3.3-6.6)	Hudson et al. (1984)

Table 11 (contd).

Bobwhite quail (Colinus virginianus)	mature	oral	LD_{50}	2.8	Clarkson & Rowe (1970)
Pheasant (Phasianus colchicus)	3-4 months	oral	LD_{50}	5.3 (3.9-7.4)	Hudson et al. (1984)
Pheasant (Phasianus colchicus)	10 days	diet	LC_{50}	>300	Hill et al. (1975)
Japanese quail (C. coturnix japonica)	14 days	diet	LC_{50}	387 (336-445)	Hill & Camardese (1986)
Mallard duck (Anas platyrhynchos)	5 days 10 days	diet diet	LC_{50} LC_{50}	594 (507-695) < 1000[c]	Hill et al. (1975)

[a] Oral dosing consisted of a single capsular dose. Dietary dosing consisted of 5 days feeding on a contaminated diet followed by a 2-day observation period.

[b] LD_{50} = lethal dose for 50% of animals, expressed as mg/kg body weight. LC_{50} = lethal concentration for 50% of animals, expressed as mg/kg diet. M = male; F = female.

[c] There was 70% mortality at 1000 mg/kg.

[d] Letter by E.W. Schafer, Jr, dated 28 April 1975: Summary of three data sheets on avian toxicity. Union Carbide Agricultural Products Company.

second dose, and the remaining three chickens died after the third dose (day 3).

Farage-Elawar et al. (1988) compared the sensitivity of young and adult chickens to aldicarb and carbaryl. Brain, liver, and plasma cholinesterase levels were measured and histological examinations were conducted. Adult chickens showed no changes in any of the parameters measured. Brain acetylcholinesterase, plasma cholinesterase, plasma carboxylesterase, and liver cholinesterase were all inhibited in young chickens, but there were no histological changes or alterations in neurotoxic esterase or liver carboxylesterase in the young birds.

In a study by Belal et al. (1983), aldicarb was administered in the feed of 1-week-old chickens at a dietary level of 1 mg/kg. After 11 days of treatment, the mortality rate was 27%. Blood cholinesterase activity levels were reduced by 74.3% during this treatment period.

Spierenburg et al. (1985) reported that six cows became ill and two died after the accidental spill of Temik in a pasture. Chemical analyses for aldicarb in the rumen of one of the dead animals revealed the presence of aldicarb at a concentration above the lethal dose. Examination for aldicarb residues showed the meat and organs to be unfit for human consumption.

Schafer & Bowles (1985) found the approximate acute oral LD_{50} of aldicarb for the deermouse *Peromyscus maniculatus* to be 1-6 mg/kg body weight.

9.4 Population and ecosystem effects

No studies have revealed effects at the population level resulting from the recommended use of the pesticide aldicarb, nor has significant introduction of aldicarb or its metabolites into the food chain been reported in the limited information available (Woodham et al., 1973b).

Of 48 bobwhite quail (*Colinus virginianus*) penned in treated fields (34 kg/ha), only one died as a result of ingesting Temik 10G granules. No effects were seen on the body weight of the test birds compared to controls (Clarkson et al., 1968). In a second study, Clarkson (1968a) misapplied Temik 10G to fields by surface broadcast or "spilled" it in one corner of the pen as a small heap of granules. No deaths of bobwhite quail were seen in the broadcast application, but the birds consumed "spilled" granules and died. Chickens refused to eat "spilled" granules even when hungry. Further studies were reviewed by Clarkson et al. (1969) who concluded that broadcast Temik 10G granules could be toxic to bobwhite quail in the field under conditions of confinement and food stress. Incorporation of the granules into the soil and/or irrigation reduced or eliminated the potential hazard.

In a study in which Woodham et al. (1973b) examined total toxic aldicarb residues in weeds, grasses, and wildlife in Texas after the soil was treated with aldicarb, no evidence of mortality among mammal or bird populations was observed in treated or adjacent areas. Of the small mammals, coyotes, and birds examined, only one bird had detectable levels of aldicarb residues (an oriole with a concentration level of 0.07 mg/kg). In all, 8 mammals and 14 birds were sampled.

Bunyan et al. (1981) conducted an extensive field trial with sampling of invertebrates, birds, and small mammals around fields of sugar beet treated in furrow with aldicarb granules (10% ai) at 1.12 kg aldicarb per ha. A dead partridge and high levels of residues in blackbirds and two small mammals trapped within the treated field indicated to the authors that the most significant hazard of aldicarb was from direct ingestion of non-incorporated granules by ground feeders soon after application. A secondary hazard involved aldicarb-poisoned earthworms that came to the surface of the soil particularly in wet conditions. Moribund worms containing residues were found 2-6 days after drilling. Low residues of aldicarb were found in herbivores eating young plants that had systemically absorbed aldicarb. Residues and reduced esterase activity in brain were found in a number of bird species feeding on the ground, indicating that exposure to aldicarb can be widespread in the case of granular application.

The death of 600 songbirds, poisoned following the surface application of Temik granules without incorporation into the soil was reported by Baron & Merrian (1988).

10. EVALUATION OF HUMAN HEALTH RISKS AND EFFECTS ON THE ENVIRONMENT

10.1 Evaluation of human health risks

Aldicarb is an extremely hazardous pesticide. The human health risk arises mainly from the improper use of aldicarb and a failure to use protective equipment during its manufacture, formulation, and application. Aldicarb may contaminate food and drinking-water. The effects of excessive exposure are acute and reversible. Although the cholinergic effects may be severe and incapacitating and require hospitalization, seldom have they been fatal.

10.1.1 Exposure levels

10.1.1.1 General population

The main possible sources for general population exposure are food and water.

Some data are available in the USA to estimate daily dietary intake of aldicarb (see section 5.2). Extensive data show that residues in most harvested crops are generally low and do not exceed the maximum residue limits if aldicarb is used according to good agricultural practice and recommended pre-harvesting periods are followed. However, even in this case, levels up to 1 mg/kg, and occasionally more, have been found in potatoes.

High levels of aldicarb have been discovered in some food crops treated illegally with aldicarb. One poisoning incident occurred after the consumption of hydroponically grown cucumbers with levels of 6.6-10.7 mg aldicarb/kg. Two incidences of poisoning were reported in the USA from contaminated watermelons where aldicarb levels ranged from < 0.01 to 6.3 mg/kg. However, there is no certainty that this range reflected the actual exposure.

Contamination of ground water by aldicarb has occurred. About 12% of wells monitored in some regions of Canada exceeded 9 μg/litre. Of 7802 wells sampled in New York State, USA, in an area of aldicarb use on potatoes,

5745 (73.6%) had no detectable residues, 1032 (13.3%) had trace amounts, and 1025 (13.1%) had concentrations greater than 7 µg/litre.

A nationwide survey of 15 000 private wells in the USA showed levels of aldicarb in the water between 1 and 50 µg/litre in approximately one-third of the positive samples. Occasional levels of 500 µg/litre in ground water have been reported in test bores.

10.1.1.2 *Occupational exposure*

Air concentrations of aldicarb during agricultural application are minimized by the granular form of the product. However, some operations, such as the loading process, may be hazardous if adequate individual protection is not taken. Over-exposure to aldicarb leading to a tissue level of 0.275 mg/kg contributed to the death of a young worker loading formulated aldicarb. The main route of occupational exposure is through the skin, especially when workers do not follow recommended precautions and neglect the use of protective equipment.

10.1.2 *Toxic effects*

The effects or manifestations of aldicarb toxicity and its metabolites (sulfoxide and sulfones) result from its inhibitory action on acetylcholinesterase. The inhibition of cholinesterase is reversible. The clinical signs and symptoms, depending upon the magnitude and severity of exposure, include headache, dizziness, anxiety, excessive sweating, salivation, lacrimation, increased bronchial secretions, vomiting, diarrhoea, abdominal cramps, muscle fasciculations, and pinpoint pupils. There is no substantial evidence of carcinogenicity, mutagenicity, teratogenicity or immunotoxicity.

In human subjects, a single oral administration of 0.025 mg aldicarb/kg body weight produced significant inhibition of whole blood cholinesterase activity, but no symptoms. A dosage of 0.10 mg/kg body weight led to cholinergic signs and symptoms and a dosage of 0.26 mg/kg body weight resulted in acute intoxication that needed treatment.

10.1.3 Risk evaluation

The risks from an extremely hazardous chemical can be evaluated only in terms of different kinds of exposure and only in terms of the safety measures available and the degree of certainty of their use.

By far the greatest risk from aldicarb is to those who manufacture, formulate and use it. Aldicarb is manufactured in a closed system. The use of aldicarb in granular form reduces the generation of dust and the risk from occupational exposure. There have been a few accidents associated with the formulation and use, but each was the result of one or more clear violations of safety rules (see section 8.2.1). However, although aldicarb is used in granules, there can be a hazard to applicators if they do not follow all recommended precautions.

The sources of aldicarb residues in food include the legal application of aldicarb to soil in which crops for which aldicarb use has been approved are grown, as well as the illegal or improper use of aldicarb. There is no evidence of a health risk from aldicarb in food to the general population at recommended application rates and employing current techniques. However, a substantial hazard exists when aldicarb is used on non-approved crops, as indicated by reports of several poisoning episodes. On the other hand, soil application rates and tolerances for aldicarb residues have been set for approved aldicarb use to protect the general population. The success of these measures is suggested by the observation that no reports have been found of adverse health effects attributable to aldicarb exposure from commodities where aldicarb was used properly. The limited market-basket survey data suggest that exposure to aldicarb will probably not exceed 1 µg/kg body weight per day in the USA. This is well below the acceptable daily intake (ADI) established by the Joint FAO/WHO Meeting on Pesticide Residues (FAO/WHO, 1983).

Aldicarb has not been found in public water supplies derived from deep aquifers or surface waters, and thus there is no anticipated risk from aldicarb in water obtained from these sources. Aldicarb water contamination has been reported in ground water, generally at levels of

1-50 µg/litre in the USA with occasional findings of up to 500 µg/litre. However, most wells sampled in contaminated areas have undetectable or trace amounts of aldicarb or its metabolites. Reduced contamination of ground water has resulted from the restriction of use in sandy soils.

Assuming an average daily water consumption of 2 litres and an average body weight of 60 kg, the exposure of people consuming water from locally contaminated shallow wells containing between 1 and 50 µg/litre would result in an exposure to metabolites of aldicarb ranging from 0.033 to 1.7 µg/kg body weight per day. A well containing water contaminated with aldicarb at a level of 500 µg/litre would result in an exposure of 17 µg per kg body weight per day. The most appropriate available study for the assessment of drinking-water risk is a study in which aldicarb sulfoxide and sulfone were administered to rats in drinking-water. The no-observed-effect-level for acetylcholinesterase inhibition in this study was 480 µg/kg body weight per day. The estimated exposure from contaminated ground water is therefore well below this level.

10.2 Evaluation of effects on the environment

With full incorporation of aldicarb granules into soil at a depth of 5 cm, as recommended by the manufacturer, there is minimal hazard to birds and small mammals. Non-target soil invertebrates, such as earthworms, can be killed when aldicarb is used at recommended application rates. Kills of up to 600 songbirds have been reported from misapplication of the granules on the soil surface, since birds can die after ingesting a single granule. Small mammals would be similarly at risk from surface-broadcast aldicarb.

There is no indication that aquatic organisms have been killed from aldicarb poisoning despite its relatively high potential toxicity. Aldicarb could contaminate drainage ditches when used in areas where periodic torrential rainfall is likely, causing substantial run-off of both water and surface soil. However, this is unlikely to kill fish or aquatic invertebrates.

11. CONCLUSIONS AND RECOMMENDATIONS FOR PROTECTION OF HUMAN HEALTH AND THE ENVIRONMENT

11.1 Conclusions

11.1.1 General population

Aldicarb is a highly toxic pesticide.

Accidental poisoning and a controlled laboratory study resulted in cholinergic symptoms that included the following: malaise, blurred vision, muscle weakness in arms and legs, epigastric cramping pain, excessive sweating, nausea, vomiting, non-reactive contracted pupils, dizziness, dyspnoea, air hunger, diarrhoea, and muscle fasiculation. The symptoms disappeared spontaneously within 6 h. The highest oral dose that produced no observable symptoms in a human study was 0.05 mg/kg body weight, although there was significant transient whole-blood cholinesterase inhibition at this level.

The primary mechanism of aldicarb toxicity is acetylcholinesterase inhibition. It is accepted that carbamate insecticides interfere with the ability of acetylcholinesterase to break down the chemical transmitter acetylcholine at synaptic and myoneural junctions. The same mechanism of action is evident in both target and non-target organisms. There is no substantial evidence of carcinogenicity, mutagenicity, teratogenicity, or immunotoxicity.

11.1.2 Occupational exposure

Intoxication and poisoning due to occupational exposure are known to have occurred as a result of a neglect of recommended safety precautions.

11.1.3 Environmental effects

Aldicarb will not cause effects on organisms in the environment at the population level. Incidents of kills of individual birds and small mammals will occur where granules are not fully incorporated into the soil. Aquatic organisms are not at risk from aldicarb.

11.2 Recommendations for protection of human health and the environment

a) The handling and application of aldicarb should be undertaken by trained applicators.

b) The agricultural use of aldicarb should be restricted to situations where less hazardous substitutes are unavailable.

c) Manufacturing of aldicarb is a hazardous process with possible risk of exposure to toxic chemicals. Safety systems should be adequate to prevent leaks and discharges.

d) To minimize or eliminate exposure of terrestrial vertebrates to aldicarb, granules should be fully incorporated into soil to a depth of 5 cm, as recommended by the manufacturer.

12. FURTHER RESEARCH

a) Additional pharmacokinetic studies, including uptake studies following dermal application, are needed to allow physiologically based pharmacokinetic modelling.

b) A case of intoxication resulting from the consumption of aldicarb-containing mint demonstrated effects at what appeared to be an unusually low dosage. A study of treated mint might reveal a previously unknown metabolite or other factors relevant to this poisoning episode.

c) Studies of the immunological effects of aldicarb are inconclusive. Additional studies are needed to examine more thoroughly the effects of aldicarb on the immune system.

d) A reproduction study in the rat is needed to investigate concerns of fetal susceptibility. One such study is underway.

13. PREVIOUS EVALUATIONS BY INTERNATIONAL BODIES

The Joint FAO/WHO Expert Committee on Pesticide Residues (JMPR) recommended an ADI of 1 µg/kg (FAO/WHO, 1980). In 1982, JMPR revised the ADI upward to 5 µg per kg body weight per day. Aldicarb is classified as an extremely hazardous pesticide (WHO, 1990b).

REFERENCES

AARONSON, M.J., FORD, S.A., GOES, E.A., SAVAGE, E.P., WHEELER, H.W., GIBBSONS, G., & STOESZ, P.A. (1979) Suspected carbamate intoxications - Nebraska. Morb. Mortal. wkly Rep., 28: 133-134.

AARONSON, M.J., TESSARI, J.D., SAVAGE, E.P., & GOES, E.A. (1980) Determination of aldicarb sulfone in hydroponically grown cucumbers. J. food Saf., 2: 171-181.

AHARONSON, N., COHEN, S.Z., DRESCHER, N., GISH, T.J., GORBACH, S., KEARNEY, P.C., OTTO, S., ROBERTS, T.R., & VONK, J.W. (1987) Potential contamination of groundwater by pesticides. Pure appl. Chem., 59(10): 1419-1446.

ALDRIDGE, W.N. & MAGOS, L. (1978) Carbamates, thiocarbamates, and dithiocarbamates, Luxembourg, Commission of the European Communities.

ANDRAWES, N.R., DOROUGH, H.W., & LINDQUIST, D.A. (1967) Degradation and elimination of Temik in rats. J. econ. Entomol., 60: 979-987.

ANDRAWES, N.R., BAGLEY, W.P., & HERRETT, R.A. (1971a) Fate and carryover properties of Temik aldicarb pesticide [2-methyl-2-(methylthio)propionaldehyde O-(methylcarbamoyl)oxime] in soil. J. agric. food Chem., 19: 727-730.

ANDRAWES, N.R., BAGLEY, W.P., & HERRETT, R.A. (1971b) Metabolism of 2-methyl-2-(methylthio)propionaldehyde O-(methylcarbamoyl)oxime (Temik aldicarb pesticide) in potato plants. J. agric. food Chem., 19: 731-737.

ANDRAWES, N.R., ROMINE R.R., & BAGLEY, W.P. (1974) Metabolism and residues of Temik aldicarb pesticide in cotton foliage and seed under field conditions. J. agric. food Chem., 21: 379-386.

AOAC (1990) 985.23. N-Methylcarbamate insecticide and metabolite residues: Liquid chromatographic method. In: Helrich, K., ed. Official methods of analysis, Arlington, Virginia, Association of Official Analytical Chemists, pp. 292-294.

BAIER, J. & MORAN, D. (1981) Status report on aldicarb contamination of ground water as of September 1981, Suffolk County Department of Health Services.

BALCOMB, R., STEVENS, R., & BOWEN, C. (1984) Toxicity of 16 granular insecticides to wild-caught songbirds. Bull. environ. Contam. Toxicol., 33: 302-307.

BARON, R.L. & MARRIAM, T. (1988) Toxicology of aldicarb. Rev. environ. Contam. Toxicol. 105: 1-69.

BELAL, M., RIAD, S., EL-HUSSEINY, O., & AWAAD, M. (1983) The toxicity of some insecticides to Fayoumi chicks. Egypt. J. anim. Prod., 22: 127-131.

BERG, G.L., ed. (1981) Farm chemicals handbook, Willoughby, Ohio, Meister Publishing Co., p. C326.

BLACK, A.L., CHIU, Y.C., FAHMY, M.A.H., & FUKUTO, T.R. (1973) Selective toxicity of N-sulfenylated derivatives of insecticidal methylcarbamate esters. J. agric. food Chem., 21: 747-751.

BLEVINS, D., LIJINSKY, W., & REGAN, J.D. (1977) Nitrosated methylcarbamate insecticides: Effect on the DNA of human cells. Mutat. Res., 44: 1-7.

BOWMAN, B.W. (1988) Mobility and persistence of metolachlor and aldicarb in field lysimeters. J. environ. Qual., 17(4): 689-694.

BULL, D.L. (1968) Metabolism of UC-21149 [2-methyl-2-(methylthio)propionaldehyde O-(methylcarbamoyl)oxime] in cotton plants and soil in the field. J. econ. Entomol., 61: 1598-1602.

BULL, D.L., LINDQUIST, D.A., & COPPEDGE, J.R. (1967) Metabolism of 2-methyl-2(methylthio)propionaldehyde O-(methylcarbamoyl)oxime in insects. J. agric. food Chem., 15: 610- 616.

BULL, D.L., STOKES, R.A., COPPEDGE, J.R., & RIDGWAY, R.L. (1970) Further studies of the fate of aldicarb in soil. J. econ. Entomol., 63: 1283-1289.

BUNYAN, P.J., VAN DEN HEUVEL, M.J., STANLEY, P.I., & WRIGHT, E.N. (1981) An intensive field trial and a multi-site surveillance exercise on the use of aldicarb to investigate methods for the assessment of possible environmental hazards presented by new pesticides. Agro Ecosyst., 7: 239-262.

CAIRNS, T., SIEGMUND, E.G., & SAVAGE, T.S. (1984) Persistence and metabolism of aldicarb in fresh potatoes. Bull. environ. Contam. Toxicol., 32: 274-281.

CAMBON, C., DECLUME, C., & DERACHE, R. (1979) Effect of the insecticidal carbamate derivatives (carbofuran, primicarb, aldicarb) in the activity of acetylcholinesterase in tissues from pregnant rats and fetuses. Toxicol. appl. Pharmacol., 49: 203-208.

CAMBON, C., DECLUME, C., & DERACHE, R. (1980) Foetal and maternal rat brain acetylcholinesterase: Isoenzymes changes following insecticidal carbamate derivatives poisoning. Arch. Toxicol., 45: 257-262.

CARPENTER, C.P. & SMYTH, H.F. (1965) Recapitulation of pharmacodynamic and acute toxicity studies on Temik (Unpublished Mellon Institute Report No. 28-78).

CARPENTER, C.P. & SMYTH, H.F. (1966) Temik 10G. 15-Day dermal applications to rabbits (Unpublished Mellon Institute Report No. 29-80).

CDC (CENTERS FOR DISEASE CONTROL) (1979) Epidemiologic notes and reports: Suspected carbamate intoxications - Nebraska. Morb. Mortal. wkly Rep., 28: 133-134.

References

CHAPUT, D. (1988) Simplified multiresidue method for liquid chromatographic determination of N-methyl carbamate insecticides in fruit and vegetables J. Assoc. Off. Anal. Chem., 71(3): 542-546.

CID, M.G. & MATOS, E. (1984) Induction of sister-chromatid exchanges in cultered human lymphocytes by aldicarb, a carbamate pesticide. Mutat. Res., 138: 175-179.

CID, M.G. & MATOS, E. (1987) Chromosomal aberrations in cultured human lymphocytes treated with aldicarb, a carbamate pesticide. Mutat. Res., 191: 99-103.

CID, M.G., LORIA, D., & MATOS, E. (1988) Nitroso-aldicarb induces sister-chromatid exchanges in human lymphocytes in vitro. Mutat. Res., 204: 665-668.

CIMINO, M.C., GALLOWAY, S.M., & IVETT, J.L. (1984) Mutagenesis evaluation of aldicarb technical 93.43% in the mouse bone marrow cytogenetic assay (Study conducted for Union Carbide Corporation, submitted to WHO).

CLARKSON, V.A. (1968a) Field evaluations of the toxic hazard of misapplied Temik formulations to Bobwhite quail and chickens (Study conducted for Union Carbide Corporation, submitted to WHO).

CLARKSON, V.A. (1968b) Toxicity of Temik, Temik sulfoxide and Temik sulfone to Bluegill sunfish (Study conducted for Union Carbide Corporation, submitted to WHO).

CLARKSON, V.A. & ROWE, B.K. (1970) Field evaluations of the toxic hazard of Temik formulations 10G, 10GV, 10GC and 10GV134 to Bobwhite quail (Study conducted for Union Carbide Corporation, submitted to WHO).

CLARKSON, V.A., ROWE, B.K., & HENSLEY, W.H. (1968) Field evaluation of the toxic hazard of Temik to Bobwhite quail (Unpublished Union Carbide Corporation study, submitted to WHO).

CLARKSON, V.A., ROWE, B.K., & HENSLEY, W.H. (1969) Report on additional field tests with Temik 10G aldicarb pesticide on the potential hazard to Bobwhite quail (Study conducted for Union Carbide Corporation, submitted to WHO).

COHEN, S.Z., EIDEN, C., & LORBER, M.B. (1986) Monitoring groundwater for pesticides. In: Garner, W.Y., ed. Evaluation of pesticides in groundwater, Washington, DC, American Chemical Society, pp. 170-196 (ACS Symposium Series 315).

COPE, R.W. & ROMINE, R.R. (1973) Temik 10G aldicarb pesticide: Results of aldicarb ingestion and exposure studies with humans and results of monitoring human exposure in working environments (Unpublished Union Carbide study, Project No. 111A13, 116A16, File No. 18269).

COPPEDGE, J.R., LINDQUIST, D.A., BULL, D.L., & DOROUGH, H.W. (1967) Fate of 2-methyl-2-(methylthio)propionaldehyde O-(methylcarbamoyl)oxime (Temik) in cotton plants and soil. J. agric. food Chem., 15: 902-910.

COPPEDGE, J.R., BULL, D.L., & RIDGWAY, R.L. (1977) Movement and persistence of aldicarb in certain soils. Arch. environ. Contam. Toxicol., 5: 129-141.

COWAN, C.B., Jr, RIDGWAY, R.L., DAVIS, J.W., WALKER, J.K., WATKINS, W.C., Jr, & DUDLEY, R.F. (1966) Systemic insecticides for control of cotton insects. J. econ. Entomol., 59: 958.

DAVIS, J.W., WATKINS, W.C., Jr, COWAN, C.B., Jr, RIDGWAY, R.L., & LINDQUIST, D.A. (1966) Control of several cotton pests with systemic insecticides. J. econ. Entomol., 59: 159.

DEAN, T.N., SELVAN, R.S., MISRA, H.P., NAGARKATTI, M., & NAGARKATTI, P.S. (1990) Aldicarb treatment inhibits the stimulatory activity of macrophages without affecting the T-cell responses in the syngeneic mixed lymphocyte reaction. Int. J. Immunopharmacol., 12: 337-348.

DE HAAN, F.A.M. (1988) Effects of agricultural practices on the physical, chemical and biological properties of soils: Part III. Chemical degradation of soil as the results of the use of mineral fertilizers and pesticides: Aspects of soil quality evaluation. Neth. J. agric. Sci., 36: 211-235.

DEPASS, L.R., WEAVER, E.V., & MIRRO, E.J. (1985) Aldicarb sulfoxide/aldicarb sulfone mixture in drinking water of rats: Effects on growth and acetylcholinesterase activity. J. Toxicol. environ. Health, 16: 163-172.

DOROUGH, H.W. & IVIE, G.W. (1968) Temik-S35 metabolism in a lactating cow. J. agric. food Chem., 16: 460-464.

DOROUGH, H.W., DAVIS, R.B., & IVIE, G.W. (1970) Fate of Temik-carbon-14 in lactating cows during a 14-day feeding period. J. agric. food Chem., 18: 135-142.

DOULL, J., KLAASSEN, C.D., & AMDUR, M.O., ed. (1980) Casarett & Doull's toxicology: the basic science of poisons, 2nd ed., New York, MacMillan Publishing Co., pp. 374-379.

DUNKEL, V.C., ZEIGER, E., BRUSICK, D., MCCOY, E., MCGREGOR, D., MORTEIMANS, K., ROSENKRANZ, S., & SIMMON, V.F. (1985) Reproducibility of microbial mutagenicity assays: II. Testing of carcinogens and noncarcinogens in S. typhimurium and E. coli. Environ. Mutagen., 7: 1-248.

ELESPURU, R.K. & LIJINSKY, W. (1973) The formation of carcinogenic nitroso compounds from nitrite and some types of agricultural chemicals. Food Cosmet. Toxicol., 11: 807-817.

ERCEGOVICH, C.D. & RASHID, K.A. (1973) Mutagenesis induced in mutant strains of Salmonella typhimurium by pesticides. Abstracts of papers, Washington, DC, American Chemical Society, p. 43.

FAO/WHO (1980) Pesticide residues in food. 1979 Report of the Joint Meeting of the FAO Panel of Experts on Pesticide Residues in Food and the Environment and the WHO Expert Group on Pesticide Residues, Rome, Food and Agriculture Organization of the United Nations (Plant Production and Protection Paper 20).

References

FAO/WHO (1983) Pesticide residues in food. 1982 Report of the Joint Meeting of the FAO Panel of Experts on Pesticide Residues in Food and the Environment, and the WHO Expert Group on Pesticide Residues, Rome, Food and Agriculture Organization of the United Nations (FAO Plant Production and Protection Paper 46).

FARAGE-ELAWAR, M. (1988) Toxicity of aldicarb in young chicks. Neurotoxicol. Teratol., 10: 549-554.

FARAGE-ELAWAR, M., EHRICH, M.F., & MISRA, H.P. (1988) Effects of multiple oral doses of two carbamate insecticides on esterae levels in young and adult chickens. Pestic. Biochem. Physiol., 32: 262-268.

FATHULLA, R.N., JONES, F.A., HARKIN, J.M., & CHESTERS, G. (1988) Distribution and persistence of aldicarb residues in the sand-and-gravel aquifer of central Wisconsin. 1. Relationship between aldicarb residue concentration and groundwater chemistry. Adv. environ. Modelling, 13: 59-84.

FELDMAN, R.J. & MAIBACH, H.I. (1970) Pesticide percutaneous penetration in man. J. invest. Dermatol., 54: 435.

FIORE, M.C., ANDERSON, H.A., HONG, R., GOLUBJATNIKOV, R., SEISER, J.E., NORDSTROM, D., HANRAHAN, L., & BELLUCK, D. (1986) Chronic exposure to aldicarb-contaminated ground water and human immune function. Environ. Res., 41: 633-645.

FORAN, J.A., GERMUSKA, P.J., & DELFINO, J.J. (1985) Acute toxicity of aldicarb, aldicarb sulfoxide and aldicarb sulfone to *daphnia laevis*. Bull. environ. Contam. Toxicol., 35: 546-550.

GAINES, T.B. (1969) Acute toxicity of pesticides. Toxicol. appl. Pharmacol., 14: 515-534.

GALOUX, M., VAN DAMME, J.C., BARNES, A., & POTVIN, J. (1979) GLC determination of aldicarb sulfoxide and aldicarb in soils and water using a Hall electrolytic conductivity detector. Chem. Abstr., 91: 164 (91:187828v).

GIVEN, C.J. & DIERBERG, F.E. (1985) Effect of pH on the rate of aldicarb hydrolysis. Bull. environ. Contam. Toxicol., 34: 627-633.

GODEK, E.G., NAISMITH, R.W., & MATTHEWS, R.J. (1984) Rat hepatocyte primary culture/DNA repair test (Study conducted for Union Carbide Corporation, submitted to WHO).

GOES, E.H., SAVAGE, E.P., GIBBONS, G., AARONSON, M., FORD, S.A., & WHEELER, H.W. (1980) Suspected foodborne carbamate pesticide intoxications associated with ingestion of hydroponic cucumbers. Am. J. Epidemiol., 111: 254-259.

GOLDMAN, L.R., SMITH, D.F., NEUTRA, R.R., SAUNDERS, L.D., POND, E.M., STRATTON, J., WALLER, K., JACKSON, R.J., & KIZER, K.W. (1990a) Pesticide food poisoning from contaminated watermelons in California, 1985. Arch. environ. Health, 45(4): 229-236.

GOLDMAN, L.R., BELLER, M., & JACKSON, R.J. (1990b) Aldicarb food poisonings in California, 1985-1988: Toxicity estimates for humans. Arch. environ. Health, 45(3): 141-147.

GONZALEZ, D.A. & WEAVER, D.J. (1986) Monitoring concentrations of aldicarb and its breakdown products in irrigation water runoff and soil from agricultural fields in Kern Country 1985, Sacramento, California Department of Food and Agriculture, Environmental Monitoring and Pesticide Management, pp. 1-9 (Unpublished report).

GREEN, M.A., HEUMANN, M.A., WEHR, H.M., FOSTER, L.T., WILLIAMS, P., Jr, POLDER, J.A., MORGAN, C.L., WAGNER, S.H., WANKE, L.A., & WITT, J.M. (1987) An outbreak of watermelon-borne pesticide toxicity. Am. J. public Health, 77: 1431-1434.

GRIFFITH, J. & DUNCAN, R.C. (1985) Grower reported pesticide poisonings among Florida citrus fieldworkers. J. environ. Sci. Health, B20: 61-72.

HAINES, R.G. (1971) Ingestion of aldicarb by human volunteers: A controlled study of the effect of aldicarb on man, Terryton, NY, Union Carbide Corporation (Unpublished report with addendum).

HAJJAR, N.P. & HODGSON, E. (1982) Sulfoxidation of thioether-containing pesticides by the flavin-adenine-dinucleotide-dependent monooxygenase of pig liver microsomes. Biochem. Pharmacol., 31: 745-752.

HAMADA, N.N. (1988) One-year chronic oral toxicity study in beagle dogs with aldicarb technical (Study conducted for Rhône-Poulenc AG Company, submitted to WHO).

HANSEN, J.L. & SPIEGEL, M.H. (1983) Hydrolysis studies of aldicarb, aldicarb sulfoxide and aldicarb sulfone. Environ. Toxicol. Chem., 2: 147-153.

HAQUE, A. & EBING, W. (1983) [Toxicity determination of pesticides to earthworms in the soil.] Z. Pflanzenkr. Pflanzenschutz, 90: 395-408 (Abstract) (in German).

HAYES, W.J. (1982) Pesticides studied in man, Baltimore, Maryland, Williams & Wilkins Publishers, pp. 447-462.

HEGG, R.O., SHELLY, W.H., JONE, R.L., & ROMINE, R.R. (1988) Movement and degradation of aldicarb residues in South Carolina loamy sand soil. Agric. Ecosyst. Environ., 20: 303-315.

HICKS, B.W., DOROUGH, H.W., & MEHENDALE, H.M. (1972) Metabolism of aldicarb pesticide in laying hens. J. agric. food Chem., 20: 151-156.

HIEBSCH, S. (1988) The occurence of 35 pesticides in Canadian drinking water and surface water, Ottawa, Canada, Environmental Health Directorate, Department of National Health and Welfare.

References

HILL, E.F. & CAMARDESE, M.B. (1981) Subacute toxicity testing with young birds: Response in relation to age and interest variability in LC_{50} estimates. In: Lamb, D.W. & Kenaga, E.E., ed. Proceedings of the Conference on Avian and Mammalian Toxicology, Philadelphia, American Society for Testing and Material, pp. 41-65 (Abstract) (STP 757).

HILL, E.F. & CAMARDESE, M.B. (1986) Lethal dietary toxicities of environmental contaminants and pesticides to Coturnix, Washington, DC, US Department of Interior, Fish and Wildlife Service, 23 pp (Technical Report No. 2).

HILL, E.F., HEALTH, R.G., SPANN, J.W., & WILLIAM, J.D. (1975) Lethal dietary toxicities of environmental pollutants to birds, Washington, DC, US Department of Interior, Fish and Wildlife Service, 8 pp (Special Report No. 191).

HIRSCH, G.H., MORI, B.T., MORGAN, G.B., BENNETT, P.R., & WILLIAMS, B.C. (1987) Report of illness caused by aldicarb-contaminated cucumbers. Food Addit. Contam., 5: 155-160.

HOPKINS, A.R. & TAFT, H.M. (1965) Control of certain cotton pests with a new systemic insecticide, UC-21149. J. econ. Entomol., 58: 746-749.

HUDSON, R.H., TUCKER, R.K., & HAEGELE, M.A. (1984) Handbook of toxicity of pesticides to wildlife, Washington, DC, US Department of Interior, Fish and Wildlife Service (Resource Publication No. 153).

IRDC (INTERNATIONAL RESEARCH & DEVELOPMENT CORPORATION) (1983) Teratology study in rabbits, Institute, West Virginia, Union Carbide Corporation.

IRPTC (1989) IRPTC data profile on aldicarb, Geneva, International Register of Potentially Toxic Chemicals, United Nations Environment Programme (Report No. OR 2134).

IWATA, Y., WESTLAKE, W.E., BARKLEY, J.H., CARMAN, G.E., & GUNTHER, F.A. (1977) Aldicarb residues in oranges, citrus by-products, orange leaves and soil after an aldicarb soil application in an orange grove. J. agric. food Chem., 25: 933.

JACKSON, R.J., STRATTON, J.W., GOLDMAN, L.R., SMITH, D.F., POND, E.M., EPSTEIN, D., NEUTRA, R.R., KELTER, A., & KIZER, K.W. (1986) Aldicarb food poisoning from contaminated melons - California. Morb. Mortal. wkly Rep., 35: 255-257.

JONES, A.S. (1976) Metabolism of aldicarb by five soil fungi. J. agric. food Chem., 24: 115-177.

JONES, R.L. (1986) Field, laboratory and modelling studies on the degradation and transport of aldicarb residues in soil and groundwater. In: Garner, W.Y., ed. Evaluation of pesticides in groundwater, Washington, DC, American Chemical Society, pp. 197-218 (ACS Symposium Series 315).

JONES, R.L. (1987) Central California studies on the degradation and movement of aldicarb residues. J. Contam. Hydrol., 1: 287-298.

JONES, R.L., ROURKE, R.V., & HANSEN, J.L. (1986) Effect of application methods on movement and degradation of aldicarb residues in Maine potato fields. Environ. Toxicol. Chem., 5: 167-173.

JONES, R.L., HORNSBY, A.G., RAO, P.S., & ANDERSON, M.P. (1987a) Movement and degradation of aldicarb residues in the saturated zone under citrus groves on the Florida ridge. J. Contam. Hydrol., 1: 265-285.

JONES, R.L., KIRKLAND, S.D., & CHANCEY, E.L. (1987b) Measurement of the environmental fate of aldicarb residues in a Nebraska sand Hills soil. Appl. agric. Res., 2: 177-182.

KNAAK, J.B., TALLANT, M.J., & SULLIVAN L.J. (1966a) The metabolism of 2-methyl-2-(methylthio)propionaldehyde O-(methylcarbamoyl)oxime in the rat. J. agric. food Chem., 14: 573-578.

KNAAK, J.B., TALLANT, M.J., BARTLEY, W.J., & SULLIVAN, L.J. (1966b) Metabolism of carbaryl in the rat, guinea pig and man. J. agric. food Chem., 13(6): 537-543.

KRAUSE, R.T. (1979) Resolution, sensitivity and selectivity of an HPLC post-column fluorometric labelling technique for determination of carbamate insecticides. J. Chromatogr., 185(1): 615-624.

KRAUSE, R.T. (1980) Resolution, sensitivity and selectivity of HPLC-post column fluorometric labelling technique for determination of carbamate insecticides Chem. Abstr., 92: 141601.

KRAUSE, R.T. (1985a) Liquid chromatographic determination of N-methylcarbamate insecticides and metabolites in crops. I. Collaborative study. J. Assoc. Off. Anal. Chem., 68(4): 726-733.

KRAUSE, R.T. (1985b) Liquid chromatographic determination of N-methylcarbamate insecticides and metabolites in crops. II. Analytical characteristics and residue findings. J. Assoc. Off. Anal. Chem., 68(4): 734-741.

KUHR, R.J. & DOROUGH, H.W. (1976) Carbamate insecticides: Chemistry, biochemistry, and toxicology, Cleveland, Ohio, CRC Press, Inc., pp. 2-6, 103-112, 187-190, 211-213, 219-229.

KUSESKE, D.W., FUNK, B.R., & SCHULTZ, J.T. (1974) Effects and persistence of Baygon (propoxur) and Temik (aldicarb) insecticides in soil. Plant Soil, 41: 255-269.

LAFRANCE, P., AIT-SSI, L., BANTON, O., CAMPBELL, P.G.C., & VILLENEUVE, J.P. (1988) Sorption of the pesticide aldicarb by soil: Its mobility through a saturated medium in the presence of dissolved organic matter. Water Pollut. Res. J. Can., 23(2): 253-269.

LANDAU, M. & TUCKER, J.W. (1984) Acute toxicity of EDB and Aldicarb to young of two estuarine fish species. Bull. environ. Contam. Toxicol., 33: 127-132.

References

LASKI, R.R. & VANNELLI, J.J. (1984) Survey of potatoes grown in New York state for aldicarb residues. Bull. environ. Contam. Toxicol., 32: 116-118.

LEE, M.H. & RANSDELL, J.F. (1984) A farmworker death due to pesticide toxicity: a case report. J. Toxicol. environ. Health, 14: 239-246.

LEMLEY, A.T. & ZHONG, W.Z. (1983) Kinetics of aqueous base and acid hydrolysis of aldicarb, aldicarb sulfoxide and aldicarb sulfone. J. environ. Sci. Health, B18: 189-206.

LEMLEY, A.T., WAGNET, R.T., & ZHONG, W.Z. (1988) Sorption and degradation of aldicarb and its oxidation products in a soil-water flow system as a function of pH and temperature. J. environ. Qual., 17(3): 408-414.

LIGHTFOOT, E.N. & THORNE, P.S. (1987) Laboratory studies on mechanisms for the degradation of aldicarb, aldicarb sulfoxide and aldicarb sulfone Environ. Toxicol. Chem., 6: 337-394.

LIJINSKY, W. & SCHMAHL, D. (1978) Carcinogenicity of N-nitroso derivatives of N-methylcarbamate insecticides in rats. Ecotoxicol. environ. Saf., 2: 413-419.

LORBER, M.N., COHEN, S.Z., NOVEN, S.E., & DEBUCHANANNE, G.D. (1989) Focus: A national evaluation of the leaching potential of aldicarb: Part I - An integrated assessment methodology. Groundwater monit. Rep., Fall 1989: 109-125.

LORBER, M., COHEN, S. & DEBUCHANNE (1990) Focus: A national evaluation of the leaching potential of aldicarb: Part II - An evaluation of groundwater monitoring data. Groundwater monit. Rep., Winter 1990: 127-141.

MAIBACH, H.I., FELDMAN, R.J., MILBY, T.H., & SERAT, W.F. (1971) Regional variation in percutaneous penetration in man. Arch. environ. Health, 23: 208-211.

MAITLEN, J.C. & POWELL, D.M. (1982) Persistence of aldicarb in soil relative to the carry-over of residues into crops. J. agric. food Chem., 30: 589-592.

MAITLEN, J.C., MCDONOUGH, L.M., DEAN, F., BUTT, B.A., & LANDIS, B.J. (1970) Aldicarb residues in apples, pears, sugarbeets and cottonseed, performance in apples and pears, Washington, DC, US Department of Agriculture, Agricultural Research Service (Report AR5-33-135).

MARSHALL, E. (1985) The rise and decline of Temik. Science, 229: 1369-1371.

MARSHALL, T.C. & DOROUGH, H.W. (1979) Biliary excretion of carbamate insecticides in the rat. Pestic. Biochem. Physiol., 11: 56-63.

MARTIN, A.D., NORMAN, G., STANLEY, P.I., & WESTLAKE, G.E. (1981) Use of reactivation techniques for the differential diagnosis of organophosphorus and carbamate pesticide poisoning in birds. Bull. environ. Contam. Toxicol., 26: 775-780.

MARTIN, G., MAGRUDER, L., PATRICK, K., VAIL, M., SCHUETTE, W., KELLER, R., MUIRHEAD, K., HORAN, P., & GRAINICK, H. (1985) Normal human blood density gradient lymphocytes subset analysis. 1. An interlaboratory flow cytometric comparison of 85 normal adults. Am. J. Hematol., 20: 41-52.

MARTIN, H. & WORTHING, C.R., ed. (1977) Pesticide manual, Croydon, British Crop Protection Council, p. 6.

MAYER, F.L. (1987) Acute toxicity handbook of chemicals to estuarine organisms, Gulf Breeze, Florida, US Environmental Protection Agency, Environmental Research Laboratory, 14 pp (Unpublished report).

MAYER, F.L. & ELLERSIECK, M.R. (1986) Manual of acute toxicity: interpretation and data base for 410 chemicals and 66 species of freshwater animals, Washington, DC, US Department of Interior, Fish and Wildlife Service, 9 pp (Report No. 160).

METCALF, R.L., FUKUTO, T.R., COLLINS, C., BORCK, K., BURK, J., REYNOLDS, H.T., & OSMAN, M.F. (1966) Metabolism of 2-methyl-2-(methylthio)-propianaldehyde O-(methylcarbamoyl)oxime in plant and insect. J. agric. food Chem., 14: 579-584.

MILLER, W.L., DAVIDSON, J.M., FORAN, J.A., MOYE, H.A., & SPANGLER, D.P. (1985) Peer Review Committee Report - The Florida Temik study: Groundwater monitoring, Las Vegas, NV, US Environmental Protection Agency (Final report) (EMSL/ORD).

MITCHELL, A., RUDD, C.J., & CASPARY, W.J. (1988) Evaluation of L5178Y mouse lymphoma cell mutagenesis assay: intralaboratory results for sixty-three coded chemicals tested at SRI International Environ. mol. Mutagen., 12: 37-102.

MOYE, H.A. (1975) Esters of sulfonic acids as derivatives for the gas chromatographic analysis of carbamate pesticides. J. agric. food Chem., 23(3): 415-418.

MOYE, H.A. & MILES, C.J. (1988) Aldicarb contamination of groundwater Rev. environ. Contam. Toxicol., 105: 99-146.

MOYE, H.A., SCHERER, S.J., & ST. JOHN, P.A. (1977) Dynamic fluorogenic labeling of pesticides for HPLC: Detection of N-methyl carbamates with o-phthaladehyde. Anal. Lett., 10(3): 1049-1073.

MUSZKAT, L. & AHARONSON, N. (1983) GC/CI/MS analysis of aldicarb, butocarboxim and their metabolites. J. chromatogr. Sci., 21: 411-414.

MYERS, R.C., WEIL, C.S., & FRANK, F.R. (1982) Temik 5G (Corn Cob Grits). Percutaneous toxicity and skin irritancy study, Export, Pennsylvania, Union Carbide Bushy Run Research Center, 12 pp (Unpublished Project Report No. 45-88, submitted to WHO by Rhône-Poulenc Co.).

MYERS, R.C., DEPASS, L.R., & FRANK, F.R. (1983) Temik 5G (Corn Cob Grit). Acute peroral toxicity and eye irritancy study, Export, Pennsylvania, Union Carbide Bushy Run Research Center, 10pp (Unpublished Project Report No. 46-100, submitted to WHO by Rhône-Poulenc Co.).

MYHR, B.C. & CASPARY, W.J. (1988) Evaluation of the L5178Y mouse lymphoma cell mutagenesis assay: Intralaboratory results for sixty-three coded chemicals tested at Litton Bionetics, Inc. Environ. mol. Mutagen., 12: 103-194.

NAS (1986) Drinking water and health, Washington, DC, National Academy of Sciences, Vol. 6, pp. 13-19.

NCI (1979) Bioassay of aldicarb for possible carcinogencity, Bethesda, Maryland, National Cancer Institute (Report NCI-CG-TR-136).

NYCUM, J.S. & CARPENTER, C. (1970) Summary with respect to guideline PR70-15 (Unpublished Mellon Institute Report No. 31-48).

OLSON, L.J., ERICKSON, B.J., HINSDILL, R.D., WYMAN, J.A., PORTER, W.P., BINNING, L.K., BIDGOOD, R.C., & NORDHEIM, E.V. (1987) Aldicarb immunomodulation in mice: An inverse dose-response to parts per billion levels in drinking water. Arch. environ. Contam. Toxicol., 16: 433-439.

OONNITHAN, E.S. & CASIDA, J.E. (1967) Oxidation of methyl- and dimethyl-carbamate insecticide chemicals by microsomal enzymes and anticholinesterase activity of the metabolites. J. agric. food Chem., 16: 29-44.

OU, L.-T., THOMAS, J.E., EDVARDSSON, K.S.V., RAO, P.S.C., & WHEELER, W.B. (1986) Aerobic and anaerobic degradation of aldicarb in asceptically collected soils. J. environ. Qual., 15: 356-363.

PACENKA, S., PORTER, K.S., JONES, R.L., ZECHARIAS, Y.B., & HUGHES, H.B.F. (1987) Changing aldicarb residue levels in soil and groundwater, Eastern Long Island, New York, J. environ. Hydrol., 2: 73-91.

PANT, S.C. & KUMAR, S. (1981) Toxicity of Temik for a freshwater teleost, Barbus conchonius Hamilton. Experientia (Basel), 37: 1327-1328.

PAYNE, L.K., STANSBUR, H.A., & WEIDEN, M.H.J. (1966) Synthesis and insecticidal properties of some cholinergic trisubstituted acetaldehye O-(methylcarbamoyl)oximes. J. agric. food Chem., 14: 356-365.

PEOPLES, S.A., MADDY, K.T., & SMITH, C.R. (1978) Occupational exposure to Temik (aldicarb) as reported by California physicians for 1974-1976. Vet. hum. Toxicol., 20(5): 321- 324.

PETERSON, B. & GREGORIO, C.A. (1988) Aldicarb acute dietary exposure analysis (Unpublished report prepared for Rhône-Poulenc Co.).

PICKERING, D.J. & GILLIAM, W.T. (1982) Toxicity of aldicarb and fonofos to the early-life stage of the fathead minnow. Arch. environ. Contam. Toxicol., 11: 699-702.

POZZANI, U.C. & CARPENTER, C.P. (1968) Sensitizing potential in guinea pigs as determined by a modified Lansteiner test (Unpublished Mellon Institute Report No. 31-143).

PRIDDLE, M.W., JACKSON, R.E., & MUTCH, J.P. (1989) Contamination of the sandstone aquifer of Prince Edward Island, Canada, by aldicarb and nitrogen residues Groundwater monit. Rep., **Fall 1989:** 134-140.

PROCTOR, N.H., MOSCIONI, A.D., & CASIDA, J.E. (1976) Chicken embryo NAD levels lowered by teratogenic organophosphorus and methylcarbamate insecticides. Biochem. Pharmacol., **25:** 757-762.

QUARLES, J.M., SEGA, M.W., SCHENLEY, C.K., & LIJINSKY, W. (1979) Transformation of hamster fetal cells by nitrosated pesticides in a transplacental assay. Cancer Res., **39:** 4525-4533.

QURAISHI, M.S. (1972) Edaphic and water relationships of aldicarb and its metabolites. Can. Entomol., **104:** 1191-1196.

RAMASAMY, P. (1976) Carbamate insecticide poisoning. Med. J. Malaysia, **31:** 150-152.

RASHID, K.A. & MUMMA, R.O. (1986) Screening pesticides for their ability to damage bacterial DNA. J. environ. Sci. Health, **B21**(4): 319-334.

REDING, R. (1987) Chromatographic monitoring methods for organic contaminants under the Safe Drinking Water Act. J. chromatogr. Sci., **25:** 338-343.

RICHEY, F.A., BARTLEY, W.J., & SHEETS, K.P. (1977) Laboratory studies on the degradation of the pesticide aldicarb in soils. J. agric. food Chem., **25:** 47-51.

RIDGWAY, R.L., JACKSON, C.G., PATANA, R.L., LINDQUIST, D.A., REEVES, B.G., & BARIOLA, L.A. (1966) Systemic insecticides for control of *Lygus hesperus* Knight on cotton. J. econ. Entomol., **59:** 1017.

RIVA, M. & CARISANO, A. (1969) Compact dual-channel flame ionization and thermionic detector for high-specificity chromatographic analysis. J. Chromatogr., **42:** 464.

ROTHSCHILD, E.R., MANSER, R.J., & ANDERSON, M.P. (1982) Investigation of aldicarb in ground water in selected areas of the central sand plain of Wisconsin. Groundwater, **20:** 437-445.

RYAN, A.J. (1971) The metabolism of pesticidal carbamates. CRC crit. Rev. Toxicol., **1:** 33-54.

SAKAI, K. & MATSUMURA, F. (1968) Esterases of mouse brain active in hydrolysing organophosphate and carbamate insecticides. J. agric. food Chem., **16**(5): 803-807.

SAKAI, K. & MATSUMURA, F. (1971) Degradation of certain organophosphate and carbamate insecticides by human brain esterases. Toxicol. appl. Pharmacol., **19**(4): 660-666.

References

SCHAFER, E.W., Jr & BOWLES, W.A., Jr (1985) Acute oral toxicity and repellency of 933 chemicals to house and deer mice. Arch. environ. Contam. Toxicol., 14: 119-129.

SCHLINKE, J.C. (1970) Toxicologic effects of five soil nematocides in chickens. J. Am. Vet. Med. Assoc., 31: 119-121.

SEILER, J.P. (1977) Nitrosation in vitro by sodium nitrate, and mutagenicity of nitrogenous pesticides Mutat. Res., 48: 225-236.

SELVAN, R.S., DEAN, T.N., MISRA, H.P., NAGARKATTI, P.S., & NAGARKATTI, M. (1989) Aldicarb suppresses macrophage but not natural killer (NK) cell-mediated cytotoxicity of tumor cells. Bull. environ. Contam. Toxicol., 43: 676-682.

SEXTON, W.F. (1966) Report on aldicarb. EPA Pesticide Petition No. 9F0798, Section C., submitted to US Environmental Protection Agency, Washington, DC.

SHARAF, A.A., TEMTAMY, S.A., DEHONDT, H.A., BELAH, M.H., & KASSAM, E.A. (1982) Effect of aldicarb (Temik), a carbamate insecticide, on chromosomes of the laboratory rat. Egypt. J. Genet. Cytol., 11(2): 143-151.

SHIRAZI, M.A., ERICKSON, B.J., HINSDILL, R.D., & WYMANN, J.A. (1990) Analysis of risk from exposure to aldicarb using immune response of nonuniform population of mice. Arch. environ. Contam. Toxicol., 19: 447-456.

SINGH, O. & AGARWAL, R.A. (1981) Toxicity of certain pesticides to two economic species of snails in northern India. J. econ. Entomol., 74: 568-571.

SPARACINO, C.M., PELLIZARRI, E.D., COOK, C.E., & WALL, M.W. (1973) Reexamination of the GC determination of α-d-propoxyphene. J. Chromatogr., 77(2): 413-418.

SPIERENBURG, TH.J., ZOUN, P.E.F., DOORENBOS, F.W., & WANNINGEN, H. (1985) [A case of aldicarb intoxication in cattle.] Tijdschr. Diergeneeskd., 110: 555-558 (in Dutch with English abstract).

SPURR, H.W., Jr & SOUSA, A.A. (1966) Pathogenicidal activity of a new carbamoyloxime insecticide. Plant Dis. Rep., 50: 424-425.

SPURR, H.W., Jr & SOUSA, A.A. (1967) Effects of aldicarb as a systemic fungicide. Chem. Abstr., 67: 10927 (116136m).

SPURR, H.W., Jr & SOUSA, A.A. (1974) Potential interactions of aldicarb and its metabolites on nontarget organisms in the environment. J. environ. Qual., 3: 130-133.

SRI (1984) Chemical economics handbook, Menlo Park, California, Stanford Research Institute, Chemical Information Service.

STANKOWSKI, L.F., NAISMITH, R.W., & MATTHEWS, R.J. (1985) Mammalian cell forward gene mutation assay (Study conducted for Union Carbide Corporation, submitted to WHO).

STRIEGEL, J.A. & CARPENTER, C.P. (1962) Range finding tests on Compound 21149 (Unpublished Mellon Institute Report No. 25-53).

SUPAK, J.R., SWOBODA, A.R., & DIXON, J.B. (1977) Volatilization and degradation losses of aldicarb from soils. J. environ. Qual., 6: 413-417.

TAKUSAGAWA, F. & JACOBSON, R.A. (1977) Crystal and molecular structure of carbamate insecticides. 2. Aldicarb. J. agric. food Chem., 25: 333-336.

THOMAS, P.T., & RATAJCZAK, H.V. (1988) Assessment of carbamate pesticide immunotoxicity. Toxicol. ind. Health, 4(3): 381-390.

THOMAS, P.T., RATAJCZAK, H.V., EISENBERG, W.C., FUREDZ MACHACEK, M., KETELS, K.V., & BARBERA, P.W. (1987) Evaluation of host resistance and immunity in mice exposed to the carbamate pesticide aldicarb. Fundam. appl. Toxicol., 9: 82-89.

THOMAS, P.T., RATAJEZAK, H., DEMETRAL, D., HAGEN, K., & BARON, R. (1990) Aldicarb immunotoxicity: Functional analysis of cell-mediated immunity and quantitation of lymphocyte subpopulations. Fundam. appl. Toxicol., 15: 221-230.

TING, K.C. & KHO, P.K. (1986) High performance liquid chromatographic method for the determination of aldicarb sulfoxide in watermelon. Bull. environ. Contam. Toxicol., 37: 192-198.

TING, K.C., KHO, P.K., MUSSELMAN, A.S., ROOT, G.A., & TICHELAR, G.R. (1984) High performance liquid chromatographic method for determination of six N-methylcarbamates in vegetables and fruits. Bull. environ. Contam. Toxicol., 33: 538-547.

TRUTTER, J.A. (1989a) Acute oral toxicity study in cynomolgus monkeys of aldicarb sulfoxide/sulfone residues in watermelons (Unpublished Union Carbide Corporation study, submitted to WHO).

TRUTTER, J.A. (1989b) Acute oral toxicity study in cynomolgus monkeys of aldicarb sulfoxide/sulfone residues in bananas (Unpublished Union Carbide Corporation study, submitted to WHO).

TYL, R.W. & NEEPER-BRADLEY, T.L. (1988) Developmental toxicity evaluation of aldicarb administered by gavage to CD rats (Study conducted for Rhône-Poulenc Co., submitted to WHO).

UNION CARBIDE (1983) Temik aldicarb pesticide: A scientific assessment (Unpublished study submitted by Union Carbide to US EPA).

US EPA (1984) Method 531. Measurement of N-methylcarbamoyloximes and N-methylcarbamates in drinking water by direct aqueous injection HPLC with post column derivatization, Cincinnati, Ohio, US Environmental Protection Agency, Environmental Monitoring and Support Laboratory.

References

US EPA (1985) Risk assessment of potential Temik contamination of drinking water in Florida, Cincinnati, Ohio, US Environmental Protection Agency, Environmental Criteria and Assessment Office.

US EPA (1986) Reference dose for aldicarb, Cincinnati, Ohio, US Environmental Protection Agency, Environmental Criteria and Assessment Office (Prepared for US EPA, Office of Solid Waste, Washington).

US EPA (1988a) Aldicarb special review technical support document. Washington, DC, US Environmental Protection Agency, Office of Pesticides and Toxic Substances.

US EPA (1988b) Pesticides in groundwater. Data base 1988 interim report, Washington, DC, US Environmental Protection Agency, Office of Pesticide Programs, Environmental Fate and Groundwater Branch.

US EPA (1989) Protection of environment. Aldicarb tolerance for residues. Fed. Reg., **40**: 324 180.269.

VARMA, A.O., ZAKI, M., & STERMAN, A.B. (1983) Results of a preliminary survey, Stony Brook, New York, State University of New York, School of Medicine.

WEIDEN, M.H.J., MOOREFIELD, H.H., & PAYNE, L.K. (1965) O-(methyl-carbomyl)-oximes: A class of carbamate insecticides - Acarides. J. econ. Entomol., **58**: 154-155.

WEIL, C.S. (1968) EPA Pesticide Petition No. 9F0798 (Unpublished Mellon Institute Report No. 31-48).

WEIL, C.S. (1973) Miscellaneous toxicity studies (Unpublished Mellon Institute Report No. 35-41).

WEIL, C.S. & CARPENTER, C.P. (1963) Results of three months of inclusion of Compound 21149 in the diet of rats (Unpublished Mellon Institute Report No. 26-47, Section C).

WEIL, C.S. & CARPENTER, C.P. (1964) Results of a three-generation reproduction study on rats fed Compound 21149 in their diet (Unpublished Mellon Institute Report No. 27-158).

WEIL, C.S. & CARPENTER, C.P. (1965) Two-year feeding of Compound 21149 in the diet of rats (Unpublished Mellon Institute Report No. 28-123).

WEIL, C.S. & CARPENTER, C.P. (1966) Two-year feeding of Compound 21149 in the diet of dogs (Unpublished Mellon Institute Report No. 29-5).

WEIL, C.S. & CARPENTER, C.P. (1968a) Temik 10G. Acute and fourteen-day dermal applications to rabbits (Unpublished Mellon Institute Report No. 31-137).

WEIL, C.S. & CARPENTER, C.P. (1968b) Temik sulfoxide. Results of feeding in the diet of rats for six months and dogs for three months (Unpublished Mellon Institute Report No. 31-141).

WEIL, C.S. & CARPENTER, C.P. (1968c) Temik sulfone. Results of feeding in the diet of rats for six months and dogs for three months (Unpublished Mellon Institute Report No. 31-142).

WEIL, C.S. & CARPENTER, C.P. (1970) Temik and other materials. Miscellaneous single dose peroral and parenteral LD_{50} assays and some joint action studies (Mellon Institute Report No. 33-7. Amendment to EPA Pesticide Petition No. 9F0798).

WEIL, C.S. & CARPENTER, C.P. (1972) Aldicarb (A), aldicarb sulfoxide (ASO), aldicarb sulfone (ASO2) and a 1:1 mixture of ASO:ASO2. Two-year feeding in the diet of rats (Unpublished Mellon Institute Report No. 35-82).

WEIL, C.S. & CARPENTER, C.P. (1974a) Aldicarb. Inclusion in the diet of rats for three generations and a dominant lethal mutagenesis test (Unpublished Mellon Institute Report 37-90).

WEIL, C.S. & CARPENTER, C.P. (1974b). Aldicarb. 18-Month feeding in the diet of mice, Study II (Unpublished Mellon Institute Report 37-98).

WEST, J.S. & CARPENTER, C.P. (1965) The single dose peroral toxicity of Compounds 20299, 21149, 19786 and 20047A for white leghorn cockerels (Unpublished Mellon Institute Report No. 28-30).

WEST, J.S. & CARPENTER, C.P. (1966) Miscellaneous acute toxicity data (Unpublished Mellon Institute Report No. 28-140).

WHO (1986) Environmental Health Criteria 64: Carbamate pesticides: a general introduction, Geneva, World Health Organization, 137 pp.

WHO (1990a) Environmental Health Criteria 104: Principles for the toxicological assessment of pesticide residues in food, Geneva, World Health Organization, 117 pp.

WHO (1990b) The WHO recommended classification of pesticides by hazard and guidelines to classification 1990-1991. Geneva, World Health Organization (Document WHO/PCS/90.1).

WILKINSON, C.F., BABISH, J.G., LEMLEY, A.T., & SODERLUND, D.M. (1983) A toxicological evaluation of aldicarb and its metabolites in relation to the potential human health impact of aldicarb residues in Long Island ground water, Ithaca, New York, Cornell University, Committee from the Institute for Comparative and Environmental Toxicology (Unpublished report).

WOODHAM, D.W., EDWARDS, R.R., REEVES, R.G., & SCHUTZMANN, R.L. (1973a) Total toxic aldicarb residues in soil, cotton seed, and cotton lint following a soil treatment with the insecticide on the Texas High Plains. J. agric. food Chem., 21: 303-307.

WOODHAM, D.W., REEVES, R.G., & EDWARDS, R.R. (1973b) Total toxic aldicarb residues in weeds, grasses, and wildlife from the Texas High Plains following a soil treatment with insecticide. J. agric. food Chem., 21: 604-607.

References

WOODSIDE, M.D., WEIL, C.S., & COX, E.F. (1977) Inclusion in the diet of rats for three generations (aldicarb sulfone), dominant lethal mutagenesis and teratology studies (Unpublished Mellon Institute Report No. 419, submitted to WHO by Union Carbide Corporation).

WORTHING, C.R. & WALKER, S.B. (1987) The pesticide manual: a world compendium, 8th ed., London, British Crop Protection Council.

WRIGHT, L.H., JACKSON, M.D., & LEWIS, R.G. (1982) Determination of aldicarb residues in water by combined high performance liquid chromatography/mass spectrometry. Bull. environ. Contam. Toxicol., 28: 740-747.

WYMAN, J.A., JONES, R.L., JOSE, M., CURWEN, D., & HANSEN, J.L. (1987) Environmental fate studies of aldicarb and aldoxycarb applications to Wisconsin potatoes. J. Contam. Hydrol., 2: 61-72.

RESUME

1. Identité, propriétés et méthodes d'analyse

L'aldicarbe est un ester carbamique. Il se présente sous la forme d'un solide cristallin blanc, modérément soluble dans l'eau, sensible à l'oxydation et à l'hydrolyse.

Plusieurs méthodes d'analyse sont utilisables, notamment la chromatographie en couche mince, la chromatographie en phase gazeuse (capture d'électrons, ionisation de flamme, etc.) et la chromatographie en phase liquide. Actuellement la méthode de choix pour le dosage de l'aldicarbe et de ses principaux produits de décomposition est la chromatographie en phase liquide à haute performance avec formation de dérivés après passage sur colonne et détection par fluorescence.

2. Usages, sources et niveaux d'exposition

L'aldicarbe est un pesticide endothérapique que l'on applique dans le sol pour détruire certains insectes, acariens et nématodes. Les récoltes concernées sont très diverses: bananes, coton, café, maïs, oignons, agrumes, haricots (secs), noix de pécan, pommes de terre, arachide, soja, betteraves sucrières, canne à sucre, patates douces, sorgho, tabac ainsi que les plantes ornementales et les pépinières. L'exposition de la population générale à l'aldicarbe et à ses métabolites toxiques (le sulfoxyde et la sulfone) intervient principalement par l'intermédiaire des aliments. C'est ainsi que l'ingestion de produits alimentaires contaminés a entraîné des cas d'intoxication par l'aldicarbe ou ses métabolites toxiques (sulfoxyde et sulfone).

En raison de la forte toxicité aiguë de l'aldicarbe, l'inhalation et le contact cutané avec cette substance, dans des conditions d'exposition professionnelle, peuvent être dangereuses pour les travailleurs en l'absence de mesures de prévention. On dénombre quelques cas d'exposition accidentelle de travailleurs qui s'expliquent par des erreurs de manipulation ou l'absence de mesures de protection.

Résumé

L'aldicarbe s'oxyde rapidement en sulfoxyde, le taux de conversion étant de 48% en l'espace de sept jours après application sur certains types de sol. L'oxydation en sulfone est beaucoup plus lente. L'hydrolyse du groupement ester carbamique, qui inactive le pesticide, dépend du pH, la demi-vie dans l'eau distillée allant de quelques minutes à pH > 12 à 560 jours à pH 6,0. Dans le sol de surface, la demi-vie varie d'environ 0,5 à trois mois et dans la zone saturée, de 0,4 à 36 mois. L'aldicarbe s'hydrolyse un peu plus lentement que le sulfoxyde ou la sulfone. L'étude en laboratoire de la décomposition biotique et abiotique de l'aldicarbe a fourni des résultats très variables qui ont donné lieu à des extrapolations radicalement différentes sur la base d'observations en situation réelle. En ce qui concerne les produits de dégradation de l'aldicarbe, ce sont les données obtenues sur le terrain qui permettent les hypothèses les plus fiables quant à la destinée de ce pesticide.

Les terrains sablonneux à faible teneur en matières organiques permettent un lessivage maximal, en particulier lorsque la nappe phréatique est haute. Des nappes de drainage et des puits de faible profondeur ont été contaminés par du sulfoxyde et de la sulfone d'aldicarbe; les concentrations étaient généralement comprises entre 1 et 50 µg/litre, avec une fois une teneur d'environ 500 µg/litre.

L'aldicarbe étant un pesticide endothérapique, il peut laisser des résidus dans les aliments. On a fait état de résidus dépassant 1 mg/kg dans des pommes de terre crues. Aux Etats-Unis d'Amérique, où la limite de tolérance pour les pommes de terre est de 1 mg/kg, on a signalé des teneurs en résidus allant jusqu'à 0,82 mg/kg à la suite d'essais contrôlés sur le terrain aux doses d'emploi recommandées par le fabriquant. Les données obtenues ont permis de fixer le 95ème percentile à 0,43 mg/kg, cette valeur atteignant 0,0677 mg/kg dans les pommes de terre crues lors d'une enquête basée sur le panier de la ménagère.

3. Cinétique et métabolisme

L'aldicarbe est bien résorbé au niveau des voies digestives et dans une moindre mesure, au niveau de la peau. Présent sous la forme de poussière, il pourrait être très facilement absorbé dans les voies respiratoires. Il se distribue dans l'ensemble des tissus et notamment dans ceux du foetus de rat en développement. Il subit ensuite une transformation métabolique en sulfoxyde et en sulfone, qui sont tous deux toxiques, puis une détoxification par hydrolyse en oximes et en nitriles. L'excrétion de l'aldicarbe et de ses métabolites s'effectue rapidement, principalement par la voie urinaire. Il est également excrété en faible proportion dans la bile et subit donc un recyclage entérohépatique. L'aldicarbe ne s'accumule pas dans l'organisme par suite d'une exposition de longue durée. *In vitro*, l'inhibition de la cholinestérase par l'aldicarbe est spontanément réversible, avec une demi-vie de 30 à 40 minutes.

4. Etudes sur les animaux d'expérience

L'aldicarbe est un puissant inhibiteur de cholinestérases et présente une forte toxicité aiguë. Si l'animal ne meurt pas, les effets cholinergiques disparaissent spontanément et complètement en six heures. Rien n'indique que l'aldicarbe soit tératogène, mutagène, cancérogène ou immunotoxique.

Des oiseaux et de petits mammifères sont morts après ingestion de granulés d'aldicarbe qui n'étaient pas complètement incorporés au sol conformément aux recommandations d'emploi. Au laboratoire, l'aldicarbe se révèle doté d'une forte toxicité aiguë pour les organismes aquatiques. Rien n'indique toutefois que ces effets se produiraient sur le terrain.

5. Effets sur l'homme

L'inhibition de l'acétylcholinestérase au niveau de la synapse nerveuse et de la plaque motrice est le seul effet qui ait été dûment observé chez l'homme et il est analogue à celui qu'exercent les organophosphorés. L'enzyme carbamylée est instable et elle se réactive spontanément assez vite par comparaison avec l'enzyme phosphorylée. Lorsqu'elle n'est pas mortelle, l'intoxication est rapidement réversible chez l'homme. La réactivation est facilitée par l'administration d'atropine.

EVALUATION DES RISQUES POUR LA SANTE HUMAINE ET EFFETS SUR L'ENVIRONNEMENT

1. Evaluation des risques pour la santé humaine

L'aldicarbe est un pesticide extrêmement dangereux. Pour l'homme, les risques découlent principalement d'erreurs de manipulation et de la non-utilisation de matériel protecteur au cours de la fabrication, de la formulation et de l'épandage. L'aldicarbe peut contaminer les denrées alimentaires et l'eau de boisson. Les effets d'une surexposition sont aigus mais réversibles. Les effets cholinergiques peuvent être graves, incapacitants et nécessiter une hospitalisation, mais ils sont rarement mortels.

1.1 Niveaux d'exposition

1.1.1 Population générale

Les principales sources d'exposition de la population générale sont les denrées alimentaires et l'eau.

Il existe aux Etats-Unis un certain nombre de données qui permettent d'estimer l'apport alimentaire journalier d'aldicarbe (voir section 5.2). De nombreuses données montrent que les résidus présents dans la plupart des produits après récolte sont généralement peu abondants et ne dépassent pas en tout cas les limites maximales de résidus, dans la mesure où l'aldicarbe est utilisé conformément aux bonnes pratiques agricoles pendant les périodes recommandées avant la récolte. Toutefois, même dans ce dernier cas, on trouve des concentrations dans les pommes de terre pouvant aller jusqu'à 1 mg/kg et parfois plus.

On a découvert de fortes concentrations d'aldicarbe dans certaines cultures vivrières traitées illégalement avec ce produit. Un cas d'intoxication s'est produit après consommation de concombres obtenus par culture hydroponique, à des concentrations de 6,6 à 10,7 mg d'aldicarbe par kg. Deux autres cas d'intoxication ont été signalés aux Etats-Unis par suite de la consommation de pastèques contaminées, la teneur en aldicarbe allant de < 0,01 à

6,3 mg/kg. Toutefois il n'est pas certain que ces valeurs correspondent à l'exposition réelle.

Il y a eu des cas de contamination des eaux souterraines par de l'aldicarbe. Dans certaines régions du Canada, environ 12% des puits contrôlés en contiennent plus de 9 µg/litre. Sur 7802 puits soumis à des prélèvements dans l'Etat de New York aux Etats-Unis, dans un secteur où l'on épandait de l'aldicarbe sur des pommes de terre, 5745 (73,6%) ne présentaient aucun résidu décelable, 1032 (13,3%) en contenaient des traces et 1025 (13,1%) présentaient une teneur supérieure à 7 µg/litre.

Aux Etats-Unis, on a constaté à la suite d'une enquête portant sur l'eau de 15 000 puits privés, que celle-ci contenait entre 1 et 50 µg/litre d'aldicarbe dans environ un tiers des cas. Occasionnellement, on a relevé lors de forages de contrôle, des concentrations de 500 mg/litre dans les eaux souterraines.

1.1.2 Exposition professionnelle

Lorsqu'on effectue des épandages à des fins agricoles, on peut réduire les concentrations atmosphériques d'aldicarbe en utilisant le produit sous forme de granulés. Toutefois certaines opérations, comme le chargement, demeurent dangereuses si des mesures de protection individuelle suffisantes ne sont pas prises. Un jeune ouvrier qui travaillait au chargement d'une formulation d'aldicarbe est décédé par suite d'une surexposition à ce produit qui avait conduit une concentration tissulaire de 0,275 mg/kg. La principale voie d'exposition professionnelle est la voie cutanée, en particulier lorsque les ouvriers ne respectent pas les précautions d'emploi et omettent d'utiliser un équipement protecteur.

1.2 Effets toxiques

Les effets ou manifestations toxiques de l'aldicarbe et de ses métabolites (sulfoxyde et sulfone) proviennent de leur action inhibitrice sur l'acétylcholinestérase. Cette inhibition est réversible. Les symptômes, qui dépendent de l'ampleur et de la gravité de l'exposition, sont les suivants: maux de tête, sensation vertigineuse, anxiété, sueur profuse, salivation, lacrymation, hypersécrétions bronchiques, vomissements, diarrhées, coliques, fibrillation musculaire et myosis. Rien n'indique que le produit soit cancérogène, mutagène, tératogène ou immunotoxique.

Chez l'homme, l'administration par voie orale d'une seule dose de 0,025 mg d'aldicarbe par kg de poids corporel a produit une inhibition sensible de l'activité cholinestérasique du sang total, qui est toutefois restée asymptomatique. A la dose de 0,10 mg/kg de poids corporel, sont apparus des symptômes cholinergiques et à celle de 0,26 mg/kg une intoxication aiguë nécessitant un traitement.

1.3 Evaluation du risque

Les risques découlant de l'utilisation d'une substance chimique extrêmement dangereuse ne peuvent s'évaluer qu'en fonction des différents types d'exposition, ainsi que des mesures de sécurité qu'on peut mettre en oeuvre et du degré de certitude qu'on a de leur utilisation effective.

Ce sont les personnes qui fabriquent, formulent et utilisent l'aldicarbe qui sont de loin les plus exposées au risque. La fabrication s'effectue en vase clos. L'emploi de l'aldicarbe sous forme de granulés réduit la formation de poussière et le risque d'exposition professionnelle. Quelques accidents se sont produits lors des opérations de formulation et d'épandage mais dans chaque cas il y avait eu, à une ou plusieurs reprises, violation indiscutable des règles de sécurité (voir section 8.2.1). Toutefois, même utilisé en granulés, l'aldicarbe peut être dangereux pour les ouvriers chargés de l'épandage s'ils n'observent pas les précautions recommandées.

Des résidus d'aldicarbe peuvent être présents dans les denrées alimentaires par suite de l'application en toute légalité de ce produit sur des récoltes pour lesquelles on en a autorisé l'emploi, ainsi d'ailleurs qu'en raison d'une utilisation illicite ou défectueuse de ce produit. Rien ne permet de penser que la population générale courre un risque dû à la présence d'aldicarbe dans les produits alimentaires lorsque cette substance est appliquée aux doses recommandées et selon les techniques actuelles. Toutefois il existe un risque non négligeable si l'on répand de l'aldicarbe sur des cultures pour lesquelles il n'est pas autorisé ainsi que le montrent un certain nombre de cas d'intoxication. D'ailleurs, on a établi des limites et des tolérances pour les taux d'application sur le sol dans les cas où l'emploi d'aldicarbe est autorisé afin de protéger la population dans son ensemble. Ces mesures ont été couronnées de succès puisqu'on ne signale pas de cas d'effets nocifs dus à une exposition à l'aldicarbe par suite de la consommation de denrées traitées correctement au moyen de ce produit. Des enquêtes sur le panier de la ménagère ont fourni des données limitées qui montrent que l'exposition à l'aldicarbe ne dépasse probablement pas aux Etats-Unis 1 µg/kg de poids corporel et par jour. Cette valeur est très inférieure à la dose journalière admissible (DJA), fixée lors de la Réunion conjointe FAO/OMS sur les résidus de pesticides (FAO/OMS, 1983).

On n'a pas retrouvé d'aldicarbe dans l'eau d'adduction provenant de nappes profondes ou d'eau de surface et il n'y a donc pas lieu de craindre un risque d'intoxication par l'aldicarbe qui aurait cette origine. On a signalé des cas de contamination d'eau souterraine par de l'aldicarbe, en général à des doses de 1 à 50 µg/litre aux Etats-Unis, avec parfois des teneurs allant jusqu'à 500 µg par litre. Toutefois, la plupart des puits qui ont été contrôlés dans les zones contaminées ne contenaient tout au plus que des traces d'aldicarbe ou de ses métabolites. Les restrictions imposées à l'utilisation de l'aldicarbe sur les sols sableux ont permis de réduire la contamination des eaux souterraines.

Si l'on admet que la consommation d'eau est en moyenne de 2 litres par jour pour un poids corporel moyen de 60 kg, on peut en déduire que l'exposition des personnes qui consommeraient de l'eau provenant de puits peu profonds contaminés par de l'aldicarbe à des teneurs allant de 1 à 50 µg/litre, serait de 0,033 à 1,7 µg/kg de métabolites par jour. Un puits dont l'eau serait contaminée à la dose de 500 µg/litre entraînerait une exposition de 17 µg/kg de poids corporel et par jour. La meilleure étude relative au risque de contamination par consommation d'eau de boisson a été effectuée sur des rats qui recevaient de l'aldicarbe sous forme de sulfoxyde et de sulfone dans leur eau de boisson. La dose sans effet observable sur l'acétylcholinestérase mesurée dans cette étude était de 480 µg/kg de poids corporel et par jour. On voit donc que l'exposition qui résulterait de la consommation d'eau de source contaminée se situe bien en-dessous de cette valeur.

2. Evaluation des effets sur l'environnement

Lorsque les granulés d'aldicarbe sont convenablement enfouis dans le sol jusqu'à une profondeur de 5 cm, comme le recommande le fabricant, le danger est minime pour les oiseaux et les petits mammifères. Aux doses d'emploi recommandées, l'aldicarbe peut être mortel pour certains invertébrés terricoles non visés comme les lombrics. Jusqu'à 600 oiseaux chanteurs ont été détruits par suite d'applications défectueuses d'aldicarbe sur le sol; en effet les oiseaux peuvent mourir après ingestion d'un seul granulé. Les petits mammifères courent un risque analogue en cas d'épandage d'aldicarbe à la surface du sol.

Rien n'indique que des organismes aquatiques aient été détruits par suite d'intoxications à l'aldicarbe malgré la très forte toxicité potentielle de ce produit. L'aldicarbe pourrait contaminer les fossés de drainage lorsqu'on l'applique dans des secteurs où il y a risque de pluies torrentielles périodiques et par voie de conséquence, possibilité de ruissellement et d'entraînement des particules du sol. Toutefois il est peu probable que des poissons et des invertébrés aquatiques soient détruits de cette manière.

CONCLUSIONS ET RECOMMANDATIONS POUR LA PROTECTION DE LA SANTE HUMAINE ET DE L'ENVIRONNEMENT

1. Conclusions

1.1 Population générale

L'aldicarbe est un pesticide hautement toxique.

A l'occasion d'intoxications accidentelles et lors d'une étude contrôlée en laboratoire, on a observé des symptômes de type cholinergique parmi lesquels: malaise général, vision trouble, faiblesse musculaire dans les bras et les jambes, crampes épigastriques, sueur profuse, nausées, vomissements, pupilles contractées aréactives, sensation vertigineuse, dyspnée, respiration de Kussmaul, diarrhée et fibrillation musculaire. Ces symptômes ont disparu spontanément en l'espace de six heures. La dose orale la plus forte sans effet observable mesurée lors d'une étude sur l'homme se situait à 0,05 mg/kg de poids corporel. Toutefois, on a tout de même observé à cette dose une inhibition passagère mais sensible de la cholinestérase du sang total.

Le mécanisme essentiel de l'intoxication par l'aldicarbe consiste en une inhibition de l'acétylcholinestérase. On admet que les carbamates insecticides abolissent la capacité de l'acétylcholinestérase à dégrader l'acétylcholine, qui joue le rôle de médiateur chimique au niveau de la synapse et de la plaque motrice. On observe le même mode d'action chez les organismes visés ou non visés. Rien n'indique que l'aldicarbe soit cancérogène, mutagène, tératogène ou immunotoxique.

1.2 Exposition professionnelle

On connaît des cas d'intoxication professionnelle par suite de négligences dans l'observation des mesures de sécurité.

1.3 Effets sur l'environnement

L'aldicarbe ne représente aucune menace pour les divers organismes qui peuplent l'environnement. Il peut

Conclusions et Recommandations

cependant y avoir des cas de mortalité individuelle d'oiseaux ou de petits mammifères lorsque les granulés ne sont pas convenablement enfouis dans le sol. Les organismes aquatiques ne courent aucun risque.

2. **Recommandations en vue de la protection de la santé humaine et de l'environnement**

   a) La manipulation et l'épandage de l'aldicarbe doivent être confiés à des personnes convenablement formées.

   b) L'utilisation d'aldicarbe à des fins agricoles doit être limitée aux cas où il n'existe pas de produits de remplacement moins dangereux.

   c) La fabrication de l'aldicarbe comporte des risques d'exposition à des substances chimiques toxiques. Les systèmes de sécurité doivent empêcher toute fuite ou décharge accidentelle.

   d) Pour réduire au minimum ou éliminer l'exposition des vertébrés à l'aldicarbe, il faut que les granulés soient bien enfouis dans le sol jusqu'à une profondeur de 5 cm, ainsi que le recommande le fabricant.

RECHERCHES A EFFECTUER

a) Des études pharmacocinétiques - comportant notamment une étude de la fixation du produit après application cutanée - sont nécessaires pour permettre une modélisation pharmacocinétique fondée sur des données physiologiques.

b) Dans un cas d'intoxication résultant de la consommation de menthe contenant de l'aldicarbe, on a observé des effets à une dose anormalement faible. L'étude de la menthe traitée par l'aldicarbe pourrait révéler l'existence d'un métabolite encore inconnu susceptible d'expliquer ce phénomène.

c) Les études concernant les effets immunologiques ne sont pas concluantes. Des travaux supplémentaires sont nécessaires pour approfondir la nature des effets exercés sur le système immunitaire.

d) Une étude de reproduction sur le rat est nécessaire pour voir s'il y a lieu de craindre une sensibilité du foetus. Une étude de ce genre est en cours.

RESUMEN

1. Identidad, propiedades y métodos analíticos

El aldicarb es un éster de carbamato. Se trata de un sólido cristalino blanco, moderadamente hidrosoluble y susceptible de oxidación y de reacciones hidrolíticas.

Existen varios métodos analíticos, entre los que se cuentan la cromatografía en capa fina, la cromatografía de gases (captura electrónica, ionización de llama, etc.), y la cromatografía en fase líquida. Actualmente, el método preferido de análisis del aldicarb y de sus principales productos de descomposición es la cromatografía en fase líquida de elevado rendimiento con derivación postcolumnar y detectores de fluorescencia.

2. Usos, fuentes y niveles de exposición

El aldicarb es un plaguicida sistémico que se aplica al suelo para combatir ciertos insectos, ácaros y nematodos. Este tipo de aplicación se hace en una gran variedad de cultivos, como la banana, el algodón, el café, el maíz, la cebolla, los cítricos, las legumbres (secas), la pacana, la papa, el cacahuete, la soja, la remolacha azucarera, la caña de azúcar, la batata camote, y el sorgo, así como en plantas ornamentales y en viveros de árboles. La exposición de la población general al aldicarb y sus metabolitos tóxicos (el sulfóxido y la sulfona) tiene lugar principalmente por vía alimentaria. La ingestión de alimentos contaminados ha ocasionado casos de intoxicación por aldicarb y sus metabolitos tóxicos (el sulfóxido y la sulfona).

Dada la elevada toxicidad aguda del aldicarb, tanto la inhalación como el contacto cutáneo en condiciones de exposición profesional pueden resultar peligrosos para los trabajadores si las medidas preventivas son insuficientes. Se han producido algunos incidentes de exposición accidental de trabajadores debidos al uso inadecuado o a la ausencia de medidas de protección.

El aldicarb se oxida con relativa rapidez para dar el sulfóxido; a los 7 días de la aplicación a ciertos tipos de suelo se produce la conversión del 48% del compuesto original en sulfóxido. La oxidación sulfona es mucho más lenta. La hidrólisis del grupo éster del carbamato, que inactiva al plaguicida, depende del pH; la semivida en agua destilada varía entre algunos minutos en un pH > 12 y 560 días en un pH de 6,0. Las semividas en los suelos de superficie son de aproximadamente 0,5 a 3 meses y en la zona saturada de 0,4 a 36 meses. El aldicarb se hidroliza un poco más despacio que el sulfóxido o la sulfona. La medida en el laboratorio de la degradación biótica y abiótica del aldicarb ha producido resultados sumamente variables y ha llevado a extrapolaciones que difieren radicalmente de las observaciones sobre el terreno. Los datos obtenidos en el terreno sobre los productos de la degradación del aldicarb proporcionan estimaciones más fiables de su evolución metabólica.

Los suelos arenosos con bajo contenido de materia orgánica son los que más favorecen la lixiviación, en particular allí donde el nivel freático es alto. Algunos acuíferos de drenaje y pozos locales poco profundos se han contaminado con sulfóxido y sulfona de aldicarb; en general, los niveles han variado entre 1 y 50 µg por litro, aunque en una ocasión se registró un nivel de aproximadamente 500 µg/litro.

Como el aldicarb tiene acción sistémica en las plantas, pueden aparecer residuos en los alimentos. Se han notificado niveles de residuos superiores a 1 mg/kg en papas crudas. En los EE.UU., donde el límite de tolerancia para las papas es de 1 mg/kg, se han comunicado niveles de residuos de hasta 0,82 mg/kg en ensayos controlados sobre el terreno con los regímenes de aplicación recomendados por el fabricante. A partir de los datos obtenidos en los ensayos sobre el terreno se ha calculado un nivel máximo del 95° percentil de 0,43 mg/kg; en una encuesta sobre la cesta de la compra se han determinado niveles máximos del 95° percentil de hasta 0,0677 mg/kg en papas crudas.

3. Cinética y metabolismo

El aldicarb es absorbido con facilidad a partir del tracto gastrointestinal y, en menor medida, a través de la piel. Se absorbería fácilmente en el tracto respiratorio si hubiera polvo. Se distribuye a todos los tejidos, inclusive los del feto de rata en desarrollo. Se transforma metabólicamente en el sulfóxido y la sulfona (los cuales son tóxicos), y es detoxificado por hidrólisis dando oximas y nitrilos. La excreción del aldicarb y de sus metabolitos es rápida y se produce principalmente por la orina. Una pequeña parte puede ser objeto de eliminación por vía biliar y, en consecuencia, de reciclaje enterohepático. El aldicarb no se acumula en el organismo como resultado de la exposición a largo plazo. La inhibición *in vitro* de la actividad de la colinesterasa por el aldicarb es espontáneamente reversible; la semivida es de 30-40 minutos.

4. Estudios en animales de experimentación

El aldicarb es un potente inhibidor de las colinesterasas y tiene una elevada toxicidad aguda. Sus efectos colinérgicos revierten de modo espontáneo y completo al cabo de 6 horas a menos que entretanto sobrevenga la muerte. No se dispone de pruebas bastantes que indiquen que el aldicarb sea teratogénico, mutagénico, carcinogénico o inmunotóxico.

Se han producido muertes de aves y pequeños mamíferos por la ingestión de gránulos de aldicarb no incorporados plenamente al suelo como se recomienda. En pruebas de laboratorio, el aldicarb ha demostrado ser sumamente tóxico para los organismos acuáticos. Nada indica, no obstante, que esos efectos se produzcan sobre el terreno.

5. Efectos en el ser humano

La inhibición de la acetilcolinesterasa en la sinapsis nerviosa y la unión neuromuscular es el único efecto reconocido del aldicarb en el hombre y se asemeja a la acción de los organofosfatos. La enzima carbamiolada es inestable y la reactivación espontánea es relativamente rápida en comparación con la de una enzima fosforilada. La intoxicación no mortal en el hombre es rápidamente reversible. La recuperación se acelera mediante la administración de atropina.

EVALUACION DE LOS RIESGOS PARA LA SALUD HUMANA Y DE LOS EFECTOS EN EL MEDIO AMBIENTE

1. Evaluación de los riesgos para la salud humana

El aldicarb es un plaguicida sumamente peligroso. El riesgo para la salud humana se debe principalmente a su uso incorrecto y a la no utilización de equipo de protección durante su fabricación, elaboración y aplicación. El aldicarb puede contaminar los alimentos y el agua de bebida. Los efectos de la exposición excesiva son agudos y reversibles. Aunque los efectos colinérgicos pueden ser graves y discapacitantes y exigen la hospitalización de la persona afectada, en muy raros casos han sido mortales.

1.1 Niveles de exposición

1.1.1 Población general

Las principales fuentes posibles de exposición para la población general son los alimentos y el agua.

En los EE.UU. se dispone de algunos datos para calcular la ingesta diaria de aldicarb (véase la sección 5.2). Muchos datos demuestran que, en la mayoría de los cultivos cosechados, los residuos suelen aparecer en pequeñas cantidades y no sobrepasan los límites máximos para residuos cuando la sustancia se usa siguiendo prácticas agrícolas correctas y se respetan los periodos de precosecha recomendados. No obstante, incluso en ese caso, se han encontrado en las papas niveles de hasta 1 mg/kg, y en ocasiones superiores.

En algunos cultivos tratados ilegalmente con aldicarb se han descubierto niveles elevados de esa sustancia. Se produjo un caso de intoxicación tras el consumo de pepinos cultivados hidropónicamente con niveles de 6,6-10,7 mg de aldicarb/kg. En los EE.UU. se notificaron dos casos de intoxicación por sandías contaminadas en las que los niveles de aldicarb se encontraban entre < 0,01 y 6,3 mg/kg. No obstante, no puede asegurarse que este margen refleje la verdadera exposición.

Se ha producido algún caso de contaminación de aguas subterráneas con aldicarb. Alrededor del 12% de los pozos examinados en algunas regiones del Canadá excedieron los 9 µg/litro. De 7802 pozos muestreados en el Estado de Nueva York (EE.UU.), en una zona en la que se tratan las papas con aldicarb, 5745 (73,6%) no tenían residuos detectables, 1032 (13,3%) tenían cantidades mínimas y 1025 (13,1%) tenían concentraciones superiores a 7 µg/litro.

En una encuesta a escala nacional de 15 000 pozos privados en los Estados Unidos de América se observaron niveles de aldicarb en el agua de 1 a 50 µg/litro en aproximadamente un tercio de las muestras positivas. En perforaciones experimentales se han comunicado niveles ocasionales de 500 µg/litro en aguas subterráneas.

1.1.2 Exposición profesional

Las concentraciones de aldicarb en la atmósfera durante la aplicación agrícola quedan reducidas al mínimo por la forma granular del producto. No obstante, algunas operaciones, como el proceso de carga, pueden ser peligrosas si no se adoptan las medidas apropiada de protección individual. La exposición excesiva al aldicarb, que ocasionó un nivel tisular de 0,275 mg/kg, contribuyó a la muerte de un joven obrero que cargaba preparaciones de aldicarb. La principal vía de exposición profesional es a través de la piel, especialmente cuando los trabajadores no adoptan las precauciones recomendadas ni usan equipo de protección.

1.2 Efectos tóxicos

Los efectos o manifestaciones de la toxicidad del aldicarb y sus metabolitos (sulfóxido y sulfonas) se deben a su acción inhibitoria de la acetilcolinesterasa. La inhibición de la colinesterasa es reversible. Entre los signos y síntomas clínicos, según la magnitud y la gravedad de la exposición, figuran: dolor de cabeza, mareo, ansiedad, transpiración excesiva, salivación, secreción de lagrimas, aumento de las secreciones bronquiales, vómitos, diarrea, calambres abdominales, fasciculaciones musculares y pupilas contraídas. No existen pruebas importantes de carcinogenicidad, mutagenicidad, teratogenicidad o inmunotoxicidad.

En sujetos humanos, la administración única por vía oral de 0,025 mg de aldicarb/kg de peso corporal produjo una inhibición significativa de la actividad de la colinesterasa en sangre entera, aunque sin síntomas. Con dosis de 0,10 mg/kg de peso corporal se produjeron signos y síntomas colinérgicos y con una dosis de 0,26 mg/kg de peso corporal se produjo una intoxicación aguda que exigió tratamiento.

1.3 Evaluación del riesgo

Los riesgos que representa una sustancia química sumamente peligrosa sólo pueden evaluarse en función de los distintos tipos de exposición y sólo en función de las medidas de seguridad disponibles y el grado de certeza de que se usan.

Con diferencia, el grupo más expuesto al riesgo del aldicarb está formado por los que lo fabrican, lo elaboran y lo usan. El aldicarb se fabrica en un sistema cerrado. El uso del aldicarb en forma granular reduce la formación de polvo y el riesgo de exposición profesional. Se han producido algunos accidentes asociados a la elaboración y el uso, pero en todos los casos se debieron a una o varias transgresiones claras de las normas de seguridad (véase la sección 8.2.1). No obstante, aunque el aldicarb se usa en forma granular, puede representar un riesgo para las personas que lo aplican si no se adoptan todas las precauciones recomendadas.

Las fuentes de residuos de aldicarb en los alimentos comprenden la aplicación de acuerdo con la ley a los suelos en los que se cultivan cosechas para las que se ha aprobado el uso de aldicarb, y no sólo el uso ilícito o indebido de esa sustancia. No hay pruebas de que la salud de la población general corra riesgos debidos al aldicarb presente en los alimentos en los niveles de aplicación recomendados y con las técnicas actuales. No obstante, existe un riesgo importante cuando el aldicarb se usa en cultivos no aprobados, como lo indican los informes de varios casos de intoxicación. Por otro lado, se han establecido regímenes de aplicación en el suelo y límites de tolerancia para los residuos de aldicarb en los usos aprobados de la sustancia a fin de proteger a la población general. El éxito de estas medidas viene indicado por la

Evaluacion de los Riesgos y Efectos en el Medio Ambiente

observación de que no se han notificado efectos adversos para la salud que puedan atribuirse a la exposición al aldicarb a partir de productos básicos en los que la sustancia se usó debidamente. Los limitados datos obtenidos en la encuesta sobre la cesta de la compra sugieren que la exposición al aldicarb probablemente no excederá 1 µg/kg de peso corporal al día en los EE.UU. Esto se encuentra muy por debajo de la ingesta diaria admisible (IDA), establecida en la Reunión Conjunta FAO/OMS sobre Residuos de Plaguicidas (FAO/WHO, 1983).

No se ha encontrado aldicarb en los canales públicos de agua procedentes de acuíferos profundos o aguas de superficie, por lo que no se prevé riesgo alguno debido al aldicarb en las aguas de esa procedencia. Se han comunicado casos de contaminación por aldicarb en aguas subterráneas, generalmente con niveles de 1-50 µg/litro en los EE.UU. y con casos excepcionales de hasta 500 µg por litro. No obstante, la mayoría de los pozos muestreados en zonas contaminadas tienen cantidades indetectables o indicios de aldicarb o sus metabolitos. La restricción del uso de la sustancia en suelos arenosos ha reducido la contaminación de las aguas subterráneas.

Suponiendo un consumo diario medio de agua de 2 litros y un peso corporal medio de 60 kg, las personas que consumen agua de pozos poco profundos contaminados localmente que contienen entre 1 y 50 µg/litro estarian sometidas a una exposición a los metabolitos de aldicarb de entre 0,033 y 1,7 µg/kg de peso corporal al día. Un pozo de agua contaminada con aldicarb a un nivel de 500 µg por litro daria lugar a una exposición de 17 µg/kg de peso corporal al día. El estudio más apropiado que se conoce para la evaluación del riesgo en el agua de bebida es un estudio en el que se administraron sulfóxido y sulfona de aldicarb a ratas en el agua de bebida. En ese estudio, el nivel de no observación de efectos en la inhibición de la acetilcolinesterasa fue de 480 µg/kg de peso corporal al día. La exposición estimada por consumo de agua subterránea contaminada está, por lo tanto, muy por debajo de ese nivel.

2. Evaluación de los efectos en el medio ambiente

La plena incorporación de los gránulos de aldicarb al suelo a una profundidad de 5 cm, tal y como recomienda el fabricante, representa un riesgo mínimo para las aves y los pequeños mamíferos. Los invertebrados del suelo que no se pretende destruir con la sustancia, como las lombrices, pueden morir cuando se usa el aldicarb de acuerdo con los regímenes de aplicación recomendados. Se han comunicado casos de hasta 600 muertes de aves canoras debidas a la aplicación indebida de los gránulos en la superficie del suelo, ya que los pájaros pueden morir por la ingestión de un solo gránulo. La aplicación superficial del aldicarb expone a los pequeños mamíferos a un riesgo similar.

No se tienen pruebas de que hayan muerto organismos acuáticos por intoxicación con aldicarb a pesar de su toxicidad potencial relativamente elevada. El aldicarb puede contaminar las zanjas de drenaje cuando se usa en zonas de lluvias torrenciales periódicas, que provocan una intensa escorrentía del agua y el suelo de la superficie. No obstante, es poco probable que con ello mueran peces o invertebrados acuáticos.

CONCLUSIONES Y RECOMENDACIONES PARA LA PROTECCION DE LA SALUD DEL HOMBRE Y DEL MEDIO AMBIENTE

1. Conclusiones

1.1 Población general

El aldicarb es un plaguicida sumamente tóxico.

La intoxicación accidental y un estudio controlado en el laboratorio dieron lugar a síntomas colinérgicos entre los que figuraron los siguientes: malestar, visión borrosa, debilidad muscular en los brazos y las piernas, calambres epigástricos dolorosos, transpiración excesiva, náuseas, vómitos, pupilas contraídas no reactivas, mareos, disnea, hambre de aire, diarrea y fasciculación muscular. Los síntomas desaparecieron espontáneamente al cabo de seis horas. La dosis oral más elevada que produjo síntomas no observables en un estudio en el ser humano fue de 0,05 mg/kg de peso corporal, aunque se produjo una significativa inhibición transitoria de la colinesterasa de sangre entera con ese nivel.

El mecanismo primario de la toxicidad del aldicarb es la inhibición de la acetilcolinesterasa. Comúnmente se acepta que los insecticidas con carbamato interfieren con la capacidad de la acetilcolinesterasa de degradar el transmisor químico acetilcolina en las uniones sinápticas y neuromusculares. El mismo mecanismo de acción se manifiesta en los organismos que se prentende combatir y en los demás. No hay pruebas sustanciales de carcinogenicidad, mutagenicidad, teratogenicidad o inmunotoxicidad.

1.2 Exposición profesional

Se han producido casos de intoxicación y envenenamiento debidos a la exposición profesional por no adoptarse las precauciones recomendadas.

1.3 Efectos en el medio ambiente

El aldicarb no ejerce efecto alguno en los organismos del medio ambiente en el nivel de población. Pueden producirse casos de muerte de aves y pequeños mamíferos aislados cuando los gránulos no se incorporan plenamente al suelo. Los organismos acuáticos no están expuestos al riesgo del aldicarb.

2. **Recomendaciones para la protección de la salud humana y del medio ambiente**

   a) La manipulación y la aplicación del aldicarb debe ser llevada a cabo por personal adiestrado.

   b) El uso del aldicarb en la agricultura debe limitarse a aquellos casos en los que no se disponga de sustitutos menos peligrosos.

   c) La fabricación del aldicarb es un proceso peligroso que entraña el posible riesgo de exposición a sustancias químicas tóxicas. Los sistemas de seguridad deben ser suficientes para impedir los derrames y vertidos.

   d) Para reducir al mínimo o eliminar la exposición de los vertebrados terrestres al aldicarb, los gránulos deben quedar plenamente incorporados al suelo a una profundidad de 5 cm, tal y como recomienda el fabricante.

OTRAS INVESTIGACIONES

a) Se necesitan más estudios farmacocinéticos, inclusive estudios de asimilación tras la aplicación por vía cutánea, que permitan la formulación de modelos farmacocinéticos de base fisiológica.

b) En un caso de intoxicación debida al consumo de menta que contenía aldicarb se observaron efectos con una dosis aparentemente muy reducida. El estudio de la menta tratada puede revelar la existencia de un metabolito desconocido o de otros factores que hayan intervenido en ese caso de intoxicación.

c) Los estudios sobre los efectos inmunológicos del aldicarb no han dado resultados concluyentes. Es necesario hacer nuevos estudios para examinar más a fondo los efectos del aldicarb en el sistema inmunitario.

d) Es preciso llevar a cabo un estudio de reproducción en la rata para investigar aspectos relacionados con la susceptibilidad fetal. Hay un estudio de ese tipo en marcha.

www.ingramcontent.com/pod-product-compliance
Ingram Content Group UK Ltd.
Pitfield, Milton Keynes, MK11 3LW, UK
UKHW021310180426
11947UKWH00015B/1138